The Complete Guide to Fo Reflexology

Specific ... understand, th ... s you ... erything
yo ... STO ... ow to stimulate ... cause
rela... orresponding ... bes and
... s the appli ... gy
echniqu...
org...

By the same author:
HAND AND FOOT REFLEXOLOGY

The Complete Guide to Foot Reflexology

KEVIN AND BARBARA KUNZ

Thorsons
An Imprint of HarperCollins*Publishers*

Thorsons
An Imprint of HarperCollins*Publishers*
77–85 Fulham Palace Road,
Hammersmith, London W6 8JB

The Thorsons website address is: www.Thorsons.com

First published by Prentice-Hall, Inc.,
Eaglewood Cliffs, New Jersey, USA
Published by Thorsons 1984
This edition 1999

5 7 9 10 8 6 4

Kevin and Barbara Kunz assert the moral right
to be identified as the authors of this work

A catalogue record for this book
is available from the British Library

ISBN 0 7225 3915 0

Printed and bound in Great Britain by
Martins the Printers Limited, Berwick upon Tweed

To the reflexologists, past, present and future . . .

Acknowledgments

This book exists because of the efforts and skills of several friends. Ken Shoemaker spent many thoughtful hours editing and contributing to this book. His hard work and dedication are reflected in these pages. Our thanks to Bob Dallamore who has given us insights. We also wish to thank Dick and Charlie Schwengel for their generosity and expertise in printing and publication. We are grateful to Bea Schultz for her support and encouragement, which always seemed to come at just the right time. The beautiful typesetting was artistically produced by Betty Colvin. We must also thank Emma Seitner, the typist, who plowed through mountains of rough drafts with lightning speed. Rol and Jan Schneider skillfully and patiently photographed Barbara's original drawings from which the illustrations in this book are taken. And finally, we wish to extend our sincerest and warmest thanks to all our friends and faithful clients who have stuck with us. Thanks for understanding what we are trying to do and why!

Contents

Preface

Reflexology is more than a profession. It is an exciting exploration and a rewarding way to help people with their health. And for us, it has become a great deal more. This book is an outgrowth of that.

Foot reflexology is the study of the reflexes in the feet corresponding to all parts of the body. The feet are "worked" to break down deposits which build up in them. This is the basic theme of the instruction in this book. The premise that there is a definite relationship between areas of the feet and other parts of the body is what makes reflexology so unique. There is the sense of solidness that inspires continuing study and exploration. No one knows exactly to what degree the complex health systems of the body are reflected in the feet. We have found with each passing day that there is more and more to learn. And each day the pattern on the feet gets clearer as we observe the results of working with our clients. For in addition to the "picture" of a person's health each pair of feet provides, we are given a key into the body's system. Reflexology is a method for stimulating the reflexes in the feet to cause reactions in corresponding parts of the body. The reaction could best be described as relaxation, or a return to equilibrium.

No health system ever really circumvents the body's own systems. For it is the body that is the healer, not the therapist. No drugs or surgery are effective unless the whole body is able to respond physiologically. Many of these health systems are frustrated in their effectiveness because they are unable to treat the body as a whole. Reflexology is the exciting and effective practice that it is because its goal is to stimulate the *whole body,* to encourage the return to homeostasis throughout all of the body's complex systems. Emphasizing certain areas of the feet during treatment only expedites these results. The whole foot gets "worked" during every treatment, regardless of the areas that reveal the problems.

There was a time when we believed that results through reflexology were unpredictable and sporadic, that whether we were successful in helping a client was dependent on whether or not he or she had the "potential to respond". We have since learned that the most important factor is not "who" or "what", but "how" — in other words, proper application. The key to successful treatment by reflexology is twofold: first, it is the reflexologist's own capabilities and techniques; second, and perhaps most important of all, it is the degree to which the client is committed to being healthy (getting regular treatments and staying with the recommended self-help program).

Our testimonials about the beauty and value of reflexology are certainly not the final word. The next phase in its growing acceptance and development is scientific validation. This is coming. For now we can only push on, sharing the information and increasing the number of reflexologists everywhere. We're not flashy, we don't claim to work miracles. Any reflexologist will tell you that it's not clear why or how it works, it just works. And every one of us has arrived at that conclusion simply by working on thousands of feet and carefully observing the results. The attitude is one of offering help, of showing people how to take more responsibility for their own health. We have no intention of displacing conventional, professional medicine. We want to participate in the evolutionary process, to join in partnership with other health systems in sharing the knowledge that it is possible for every person to exert more control over his or her own health.

The reflexologist's most convincing argument is in the doing. We do not always see results right away, but getting to the root cause of any illness or disorder usually takes time. A natural system requires "peeling" back the "layers" of problems (which may have developed in response to the original problem) until that prime target is encountered. When the root cause is finally dealt with, it can be startling to see how many other problems are either helped or eliminated altogether.

This book is intended as a tool for those wishing to apply reflexology either to their own or someone else's feet. We have set out what we consider to be the basic information. There is a brief history, a completely illustrated section on the techniques, a step by step description of a treatment, guidelines for the professional, rules about many topics of concern (i.e., fingernails, lotions, instruments, etc.) and a very useful chapter on anatomy (including a table of disorders with suggestions on areas of the feet to emphasize). Writing this book has been a rewarding experience. Reflexology is a gift and we now pass it on to you with the sincere hope that you will enjoy and benefit from it throughout your life.

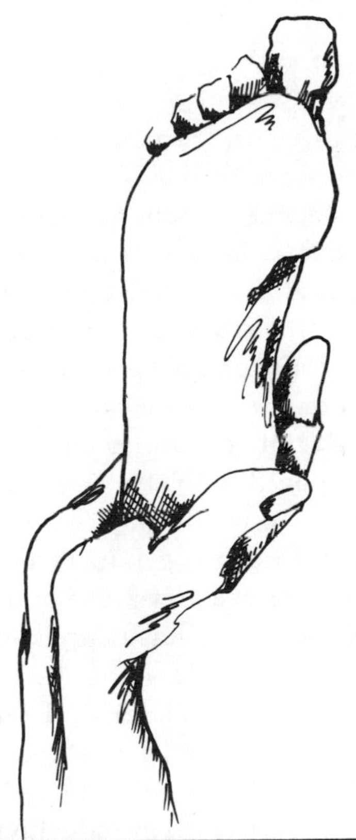

1

Development and Theory of Reflexology

Development and Theory of Reflexology

Any field of study has premises whose purpose is to tie it together into a coherent whole. Reflexology too has principles that serve to unify it as an integrated system. These principles, although simple, make a profound statement about the body and its functions. Foot reflexology is the study and practice of working reflexes in the feet which correspond to other parts of the body. With specific hand and finger techniques, reflexology causes responses (relaxation) in corresponding parts of the body. Relaxation is the first step to normalization, the body's return to a state of equilibrium or homeostasis, where circulation can flow unimpeded and supply nutrients and oxygen to the cells. With the restoration of homeostasis, the body's organs, which are actually aggregations of cells, may then return to a normal state or function as well.

One's state of health depends upon this ability to rebound to homeostasis after a trauma or challenge (i.e., injury, disease, stress). So we can say that it is the very purpose of reflexology to trigger this return. Since stress and disease are ongoing facts of life for most of us, reflexology, in addition to its therapeutic uses, can serve as a preventive program. It enables each individual, on a daily basis, to help his or her body restore and maintain its natural state of homeostasis.

The reflexes in the feet are actually "reflections" of body parts. Their locations and relationships to each other on the feet follow a logical anatomical pattern which closely resembles that of the body itself. The premise of exactly how the reflexes of the feet correspond to the anatomy of the whole body is simple: the actual physical image of the body is projected onto them. This image is organized with the use of zone theory. (A detailed introduction to *zone theory* begins on page 4).

It may be that stress is the single greatest threat to the body's equilibrium. You will notice references to this observation made time and again throughout this book. Buildup in the feet (calcification, lymph fluid) is a roadmap to a reflexologist. Wherever it is found on a foot, it is a sign that stress and its effects have begun to accumulate in corresponding parts of the body. We may *never* say it enough: if reflexology never accomplishes anything more than combating stress with relaxation, it is serving its purpose very well!!

THE ORIGINS OF REFLEXOLOGY: ZONE THEORY

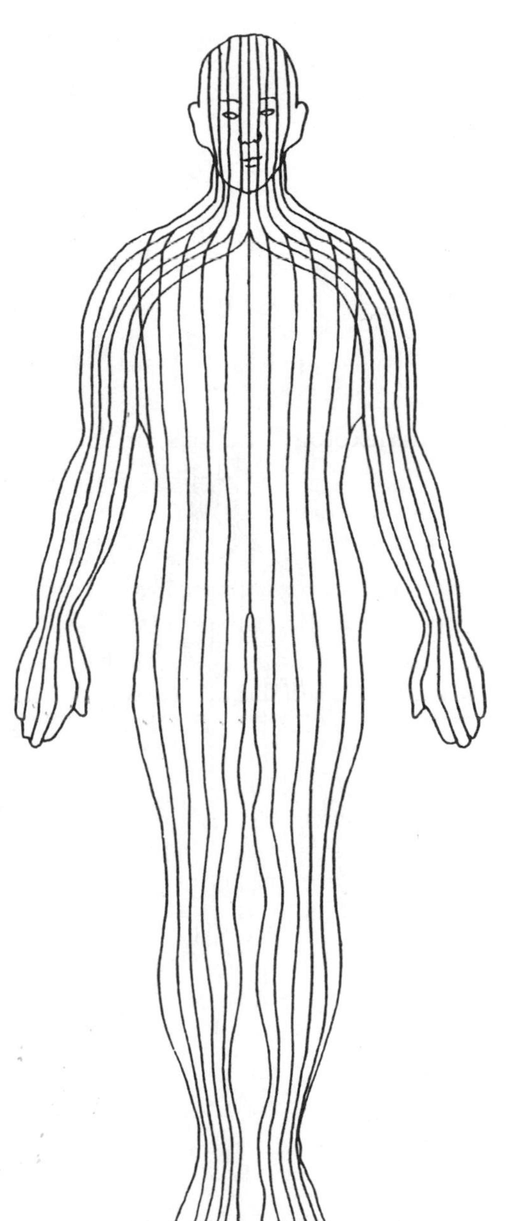

Zone Theory evolved from the research and writing of Dr. William Fitzgerald in the early 1900's. He observed that direct pressure on certain areas of the body could produce an analgesic (anesthetic) effect in a corresponding part. Just how one part "corresponds" to another is what zone theory is all about. Dr. Fitzgerald systematized the body into zones, which he used for his "anesthetic" effect and which we now use for therapeutic application. (See Illus.) He was able to deduce that his patients had been "anesthetizing" themselves with direct pressure (e.g., clenching fists) or that, in some instances, an assistant had inadvertently applied pressure. In some cases he noted that no actual anesthesia was needed before or during surgery. By exerting pressure on a specific part of the body he had learned to predict which other parts of the body would be affected, and he had taken the first major step in the development of zone theory.

Zone therapy became further popularized by Dr. Edwin Bowers. Working together with Dr. Fitzgerald, he developed a unique and startling method for convincing their colleagues about the validity of zone theory. He would apply pressure to the colleague's hand and then stick a pin in the area of his face anesthetized by the pressure. Such dramatic proof made believers of those who witnessed it. Zone therapy had other proponents, including Dr. George Starr White, who had a large practice in Los Angeles during the 1920's. Joseph Selbey Riley was another who wrote a book[1] on zone theory and continued to study it over the years.

By the early 1930's the time had come for the further refinement of zone theory into foot reflexology. One of Dr. Riley's therapy assistants, Eunice Ingham, had been using the zone therapy system in her work but must have begun to feel more and more strongly that the feet should be the specific targets for the therapy because of their highly sensitive nature. She charted the feet in relation to the zones and their effects on the rest of the

[1]Riley, Joseph Selbey, *Zone Therapy Simplified*, 1919.

anatomy, until finally she had evolved on the feet themselves, a "map" of the entire body. She must have known that, instead of constant direct pressure, she could use an alternating pressure which seemed to have therapeutic effects beyond pain reduction.

She was so successful that her reputation soon spread, primarily by word of mouth. She wrote her first book[1] in 1938. She is now recognized as the founder of foot reflexology. When she retired in 1970, her niece, Eusebia B. Messenger, and nephew, Dwight C. Byers, took up where she left off and continued her work. Much of the history of reflexology remains to be discovered and clarified. But it was its occidental origins which make it today a system uniquely its own.

ZONE THEORY

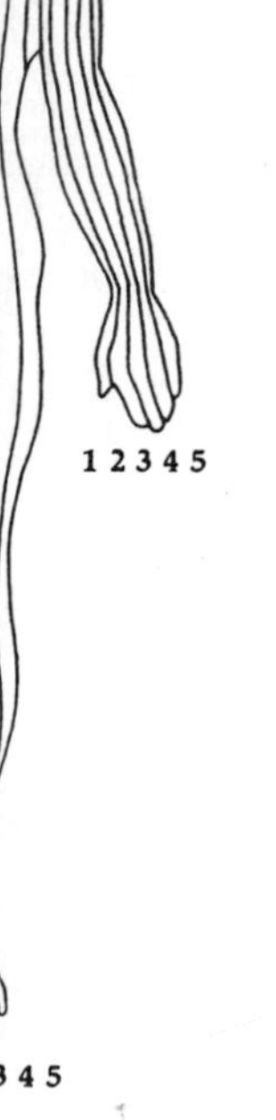

Zone theory is the basis of foot reflexology. Reflexology has become a more refined system but zone theory is still a useful adjunct to it. An understanding of it is essential to an understanding of reflexology.

Zones are a system for organizing relationships between various parts of the body. They can be thought of as guidelines or markers, which link one part to another.

There are ten equal longitudinal zones running the length of the body from the top of the head to the tips of the toes. (See Illus.) The number "ten" corresponds to the number of fingers and toes. And therefore provides a convenient numbering system. Each finger and each toe falls into one zone, with the left thumb, for example, occurring in the same zone as the left big toe, and so on.

Using the zonal chart, now trace the ten zones on your own body. Begin with your feet and trace imaginary lines from each toe up the leg, through the trunk of the body to the top of the head. Each toe represents a zone. Do the same exercise with the hands. Begin tracing from each finger. Note on the chart how the numbered zones intersect with each other in the neck and head area.

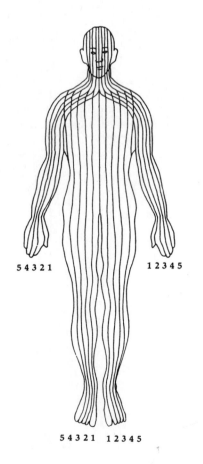

[1]Ingham, Eunice, *Stories the Feet Can Tell*, 1938.

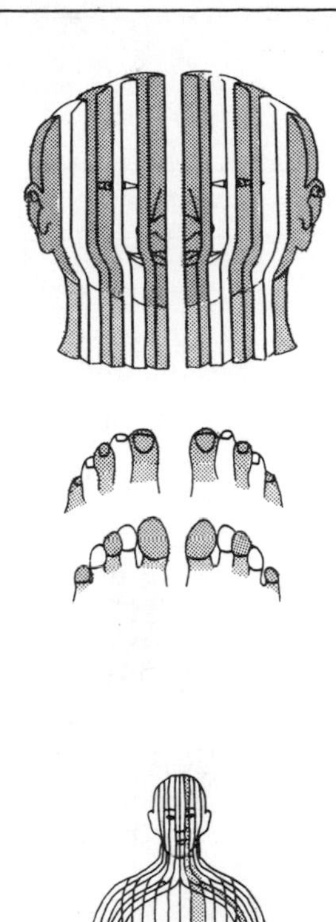

Each big toe corresponds to half of the head area, even though it also represents one specific zone as well. But each big toe also represents the four smaller toes, in that the little toes occupy the remaining zones which represent the head/neck region in finer terms. This concept is fully explained in Reflexology Theory (pg. 6).

Like an arrow passing through, the reflex points are considered to pass all the way through the body within the same zones. The same point, for instance, can be found on the front as well as the back of the body, the top as well as the bottom of the foot.

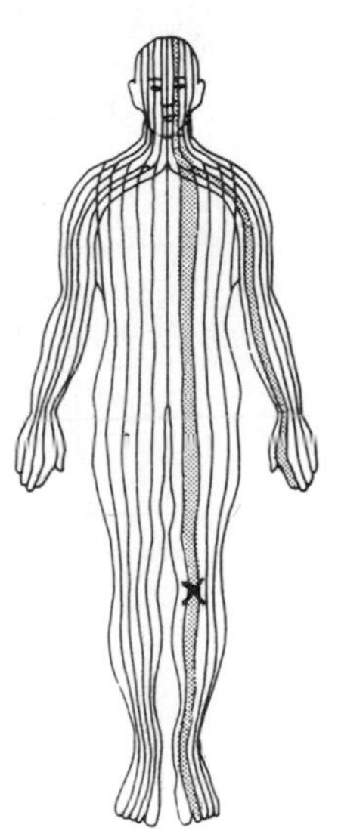

Congestion or tension in any part of a zone will affect the entire zone running through the whole length of the body. Like a river that has been dammed up, the areas on either side of the "dam" (blockage) in the zone are affected. If the area remains blocked, areas to either side can become affected. Sensitivity in a specific part of the foot signals the reflexologist that there is something going on in that zone or zones somewhere in the body. DIRECT PRESSURE APPLIED TO ANY PART OF A ZONE WILL AFFECT THE ENTIRE ZONE. This is the basis of zone theory. It is also the basis of foot reflexology. because not only are the feet functional parts of the body with representation in each of the zones, they are a direct reiteration of the body itself. They actually mirror the body (see pg. 7). However, working the entire foot affects the entire body. Because of the myriad of zonal relationships it is always valuable to work the entire foot.

There are other reasons the feet are able to serve in this capacity. They are a very sensitive part of the zonal system. Besides being "sheltered" constantly by shoes and socks, these terminal ends of the body (head, hand, feet) are particularly sensitive to the touch.

THE THEORY OF FOOT REFLEXOLOGY

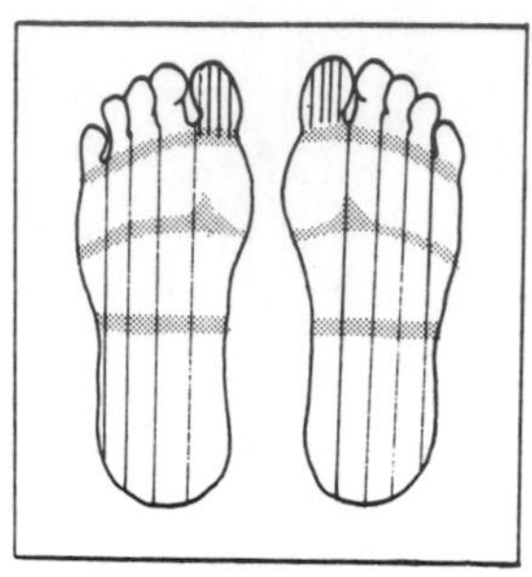

In addition to the longitudinal zones of zone theory, reflexology also uses lateral zones on the body. Their main purpose is to help fix the image of the body onto the feet in the proper perspective and location. Only three lateral zones are commonly used: shoulder line, diaphragm line, and waistline. (See Illus.) However the concept of lateral zones applies to all areas.

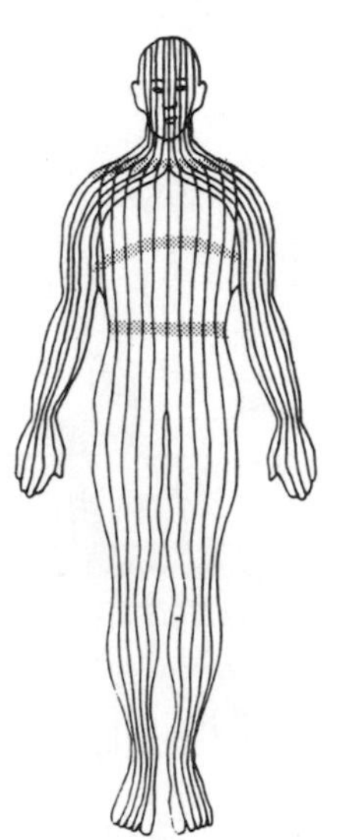

For example, consider the portion of the body above the shoulders, the head and neck region. Zone theory tells us that all ten zones of the body run through this region. As we have pointed out, each big toe represents half of the head, with the dual role of occupying zone one and at the same time representing all five zones (See Illus.). The small toes on each foot are a zonal breakdown of their respective big toe. As such, they define the head/neck region in finer terms. (The ball of each small toe represents part of the head, whereas the stem corresponds to part of the neck.) This allows us to visualize the physical image of the body on the feet. Relationships and juxtapositions of body parts can be traced on the feet as they occur in the body itself.

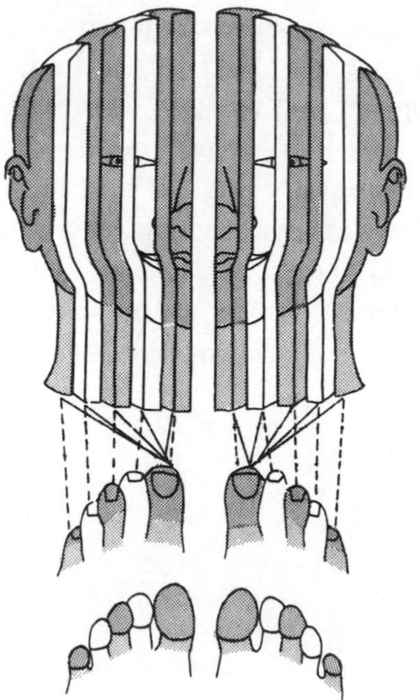

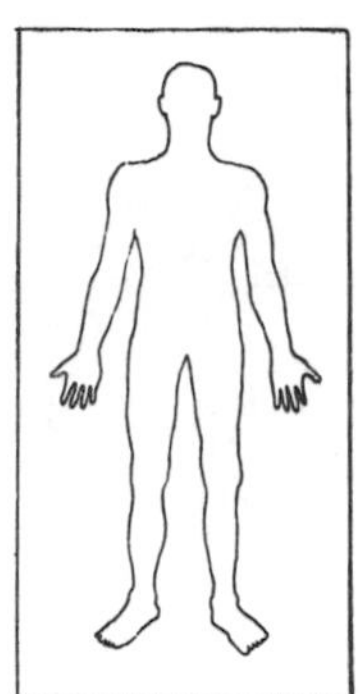

The illustration is a two-dimensional representation of the body. Even though it is flat we interpret the image as a three-dimensional one. Any chart representing the reflexes on the feet should be interpreted in the same way. Therefore, the parts of the body "projected" onto the feet (see chart) are considered as three-dimensional too. Since the feet are not flat (obvious, but we couldn't resist the pun), projecting this "3-D" image onto the feet means there is depth to the picture. We are not merely dealing with the *surface* of the feet. The reflexes actually pass through the areas where they are depicted. To help you visualize the image of the body on the feet, try this exercise: Ask a friend to volunteer a pair of feet. First, look at the bottoms of the two feet placed side by side so that they're touching. Imagine you are looking at the trunk of a body from the front. You can't see the spine from in front but you know it's there, dividing the body in half. The spine would occur "between" the two feet to be consistent with our image. But each foot represents one half of the body (right foot = right side, left foot = left side) so the spine itself is divided in half with each foot having a spinal area along the inside edge.

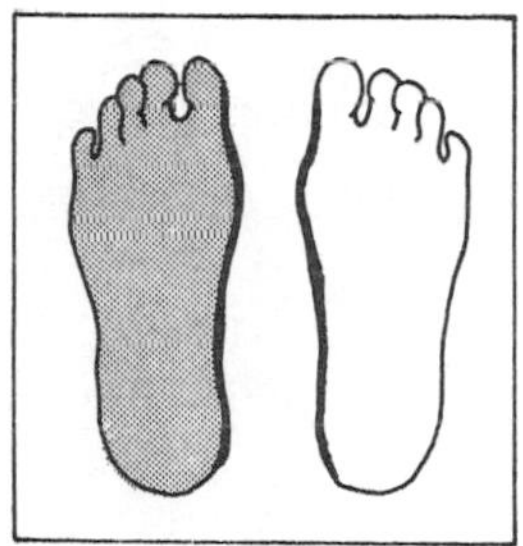

The head is the top of the body. On your trunk visualize it where the big toes are. Each big toe represents half of the head and neck. The ball of the toe is the head itself and the stem is the neck. Think of each small toe as a slice of the head and neck. The ridge at the base of the toes corresponds to the top of the trunk, the shoulder line. The shoulder joints occur on the outside, below the little toe in the ball of each foot.

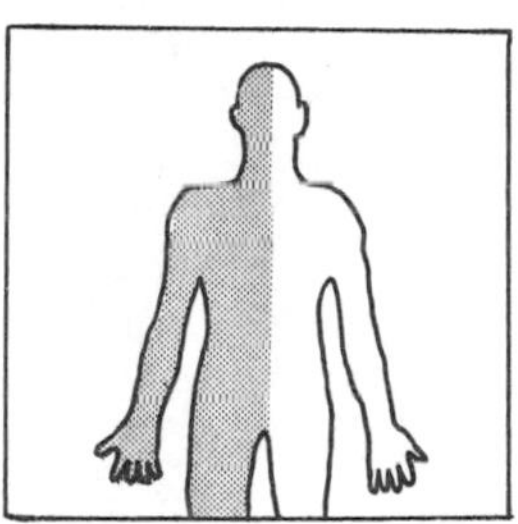

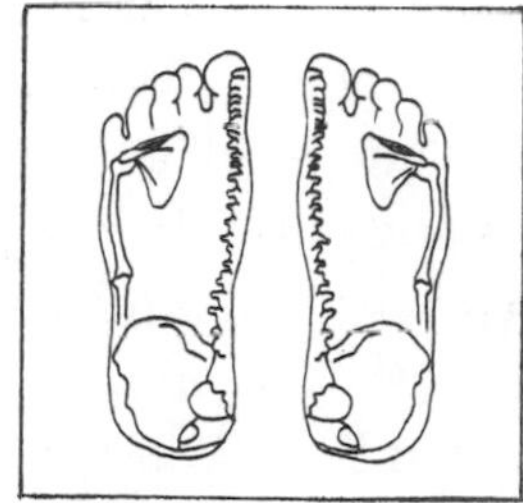

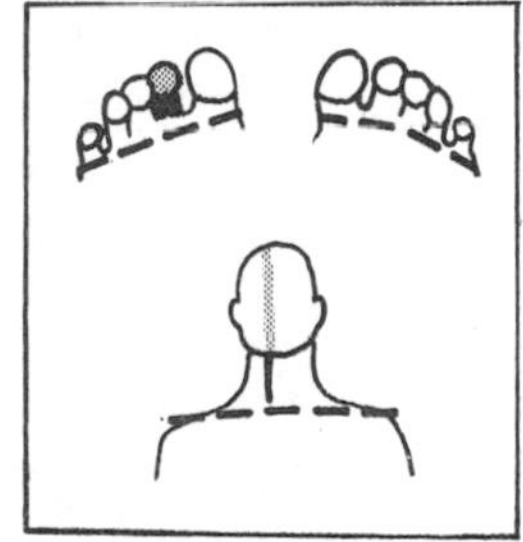

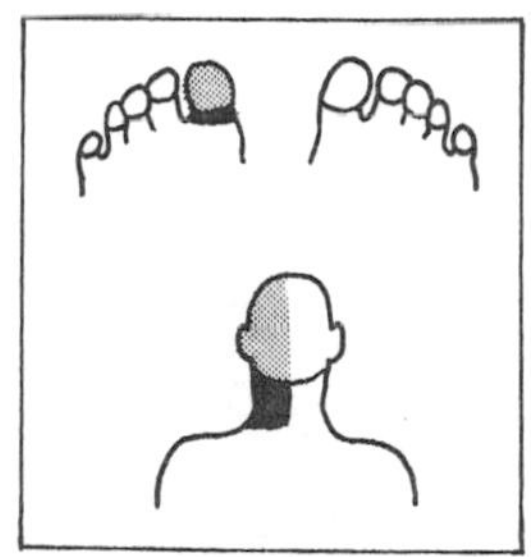

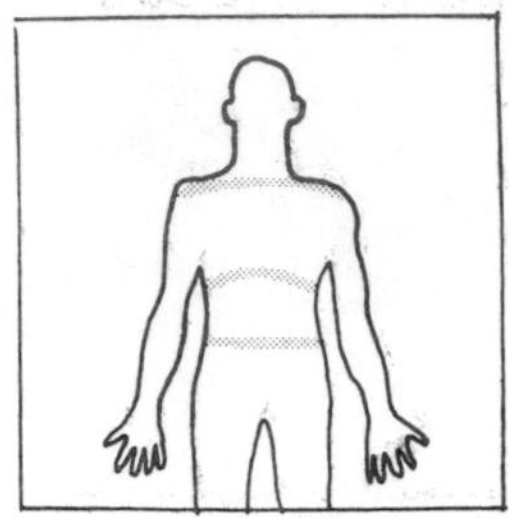

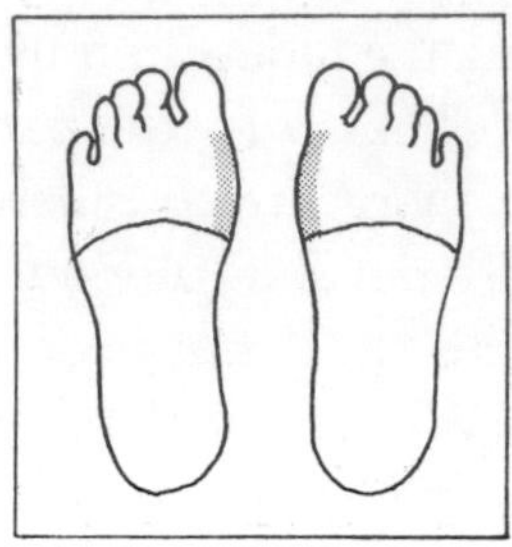

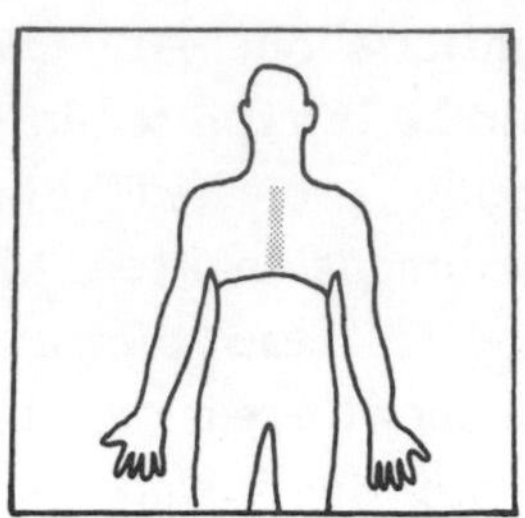

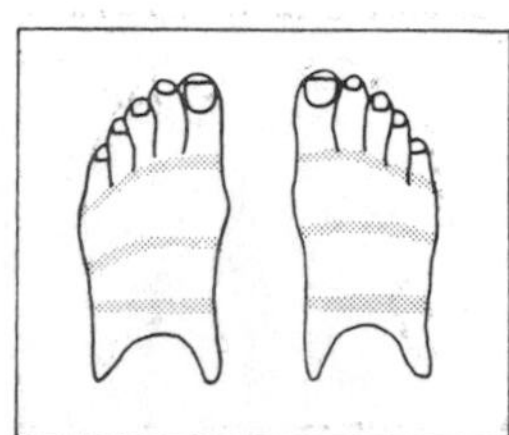

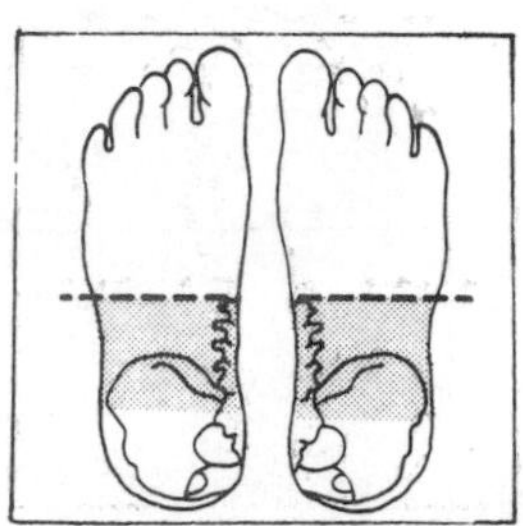

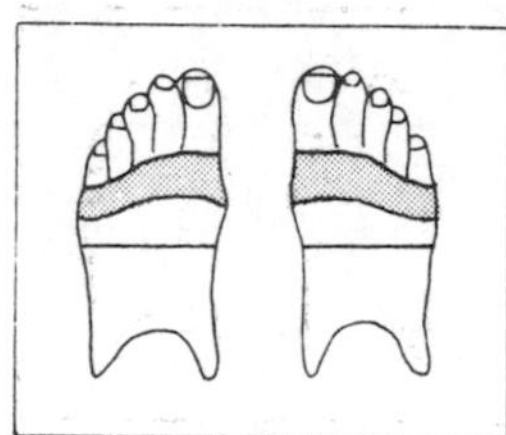

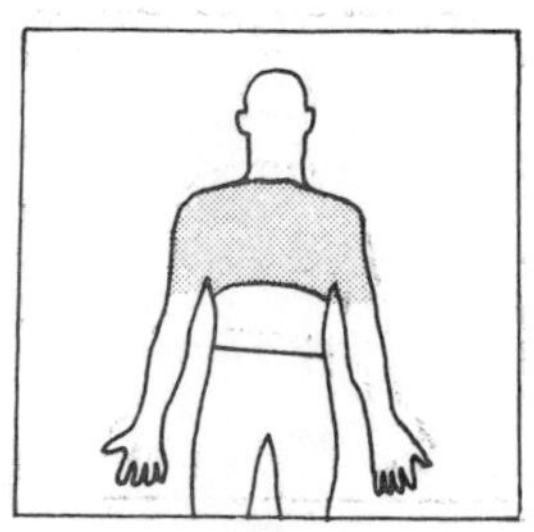

To locate the solar plexus area on the feet, first find the sternum on your own body. This is the bone in the middle of your chest connecting the two rib cages. At the base of the sternum is where the diaphragm is attached. Now add it to your picture of the trunk on the two feet. Your diaphragm line should have included the area extending all the way across the base of the ball of each foot. (See Chart).

On the outside of the foot, about half way down, is a protruding bone called the fifth metatarsal. If you were to draw a line all the way around the foot at this bone you would have a good image of the waistline. Below this line are such parts of the anatomy as the lower back, hips and intestines. On the feet the reflexes corresponding to these as well as all other parts of the anatomy below the waist are located below this line.

Next look at the tops of your own feet as they rest together. Visualize the back view of the trunk of a body projected onto them. The spine, of course, runs down the inside of each foot. The back of the head is represented by the two big toes. And the shoulder line runs along the base of the toes. Now extend the diaphragm line around from the bottoms of each foot across the tops. Do the same with the waistline, at the fifth metatarsal. These represent important boundaries and will help you properly locate the rest of the anatomy within these guidelines. For example, the area of the back between the bottom of the shoulder blades and the top of the shoulder is bounded by the diaphragm line on the bottom and the shoulder line on top. Any parts of the anatomy occurring in this area of the trunk will have reflexes on the feet between these two lines.

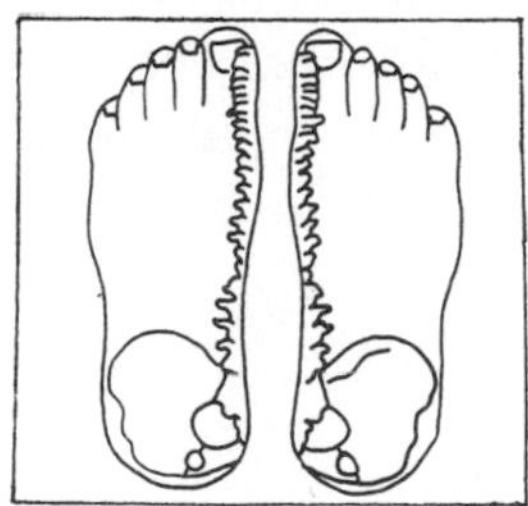

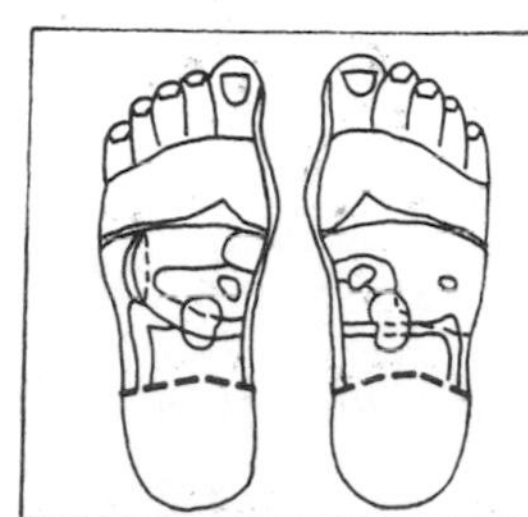

The pelvis is attached at the spine and curves around to create an area with depth (as you can see on your own body). Similarly on the feet, the area representing the hip/pelvis can be seen as three dimensional. This area curves around the foot covering the base of the ankle, around the ankle bones themselves and the sides and bottoms of the foot.

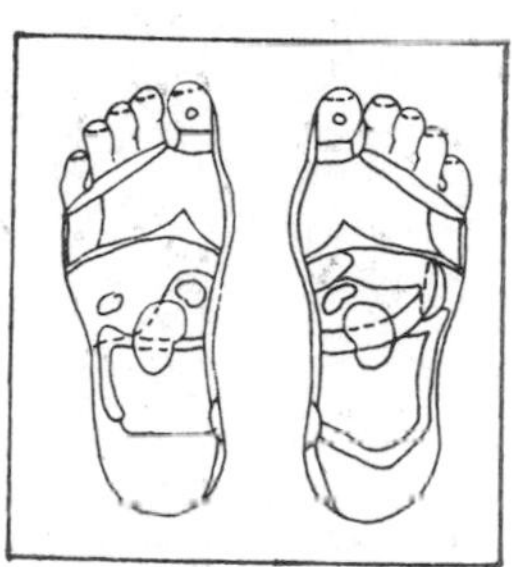

While the model we have just described is useful for conceiving the locations of the major lateral zones, do NOT think of the bottom of the foot ONLY as the front of the body or the top of the foot ONLY as the back of the body. Both the top and bottom of the foot represent the front and back of the body as well as the organs in between. In other words, the reflexes pass through the feet.

THE INTERNAL ORGANS

If you've seen standard anatomy charts in any encyclopedia or textbook, you may have noticed that internal organs lay on top of, lap over, behind, between and against each other in every possible configuration. The areas on the feet corresponding to them must then overlap as well. This is quite difficult to accurately represent on a foot chart. The heart, for instance, is more or less to the left of the midline of the body, but it extends into the right side also. There must be a small area then, on the right foot corresponding to this portion.

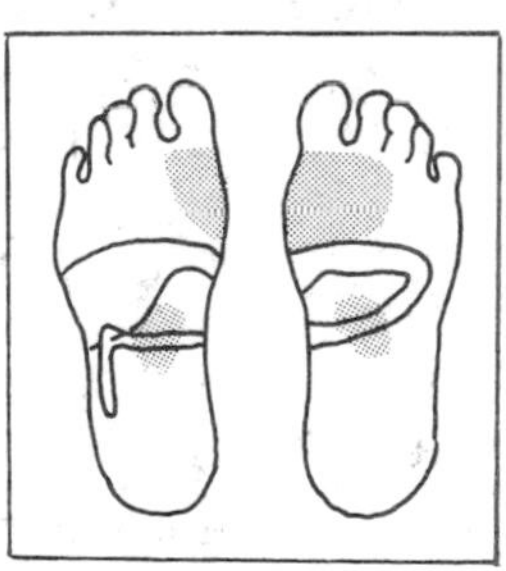

It is important to maintain the image on the foot of a three-dimensional representation of a three-dimensional body. The kidney area on the chart overlaps with many other areas just as the kidneys overlap other organs and parts of the body when viewed from back or front. Remember that the chart is designed for convenience and clarity. Once you have a solid picture of the body projected onto the feet, you will know that you are actually working through multiple reflex areas throughout much of the trunk area of the body.

THE EXCEPTION

The most fundamental zonal concept is that the right foot represents the right side of the body, and the left foot the left side. There is an important exception, however. In the central nervous system, the right half of the brain controls the left side of the body and vice versa. So in any disorders or problems affecting the brain or central nervous system (i.e., stroke, paralysis, etc.), emphasize the appropriate area of the foot on the opposite side from the trauma or injury.

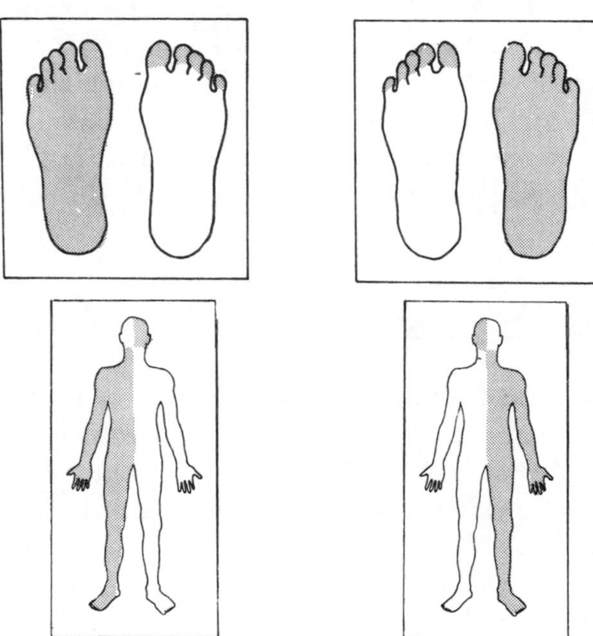

GUIDELINES

The midline refers to the line dividing the body in half from top to bottom. It is represented by the separation of the feet. Approaching the midline describes movement toward the inside of the foot (arch). Working away from the midline denotes movement toward the outside of the foot.

USES OF ZONE THEORY IN REFLEXOLOGY

It is a common assumption that the hands and feet are the only areas to which the techniques of reflexology can be applied effectively. Actually there are reflexes throughout the zones of the body. It is important to understand the zonal system because it will explain the unlikely relationships within zones. It is a valuable enhancement to the regular repertoire of techniques and applications.

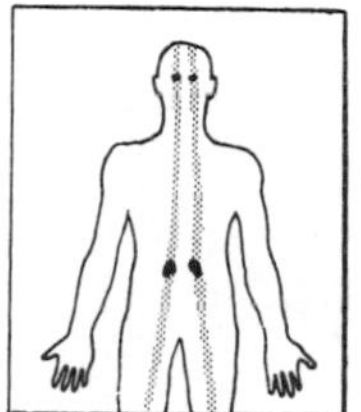

An excellent example of the unusual relationships that are revealed with the zonal system is the relationship between the eyes and the kidneys. Because they both lie in the same zones, working the kidney areas of the feet has been helpful in many cases of eye disorders.

Practical uses of zone theory include using the zones to find an area on the foot representing a pain or injury elsewhere in the body, and using a system we call "referral areas". Sometimes, when a medical diagnosis has not been possible, a *generalized* pain somewhere in the body can be traced using the zones to a *distinct* area on the foot. It can then be worked by emphasizing that particular area of the foot.

Case In Point:
One of our clients once had to rush her daughter to the hospital. When the two of them arrived the girl had sharp, abdominal pains. There was no help immediately available and they ended up having to wait two hours for a doctor. During that time the daughter was not treated, nor was she given any pain killers. So her mother took off the girl's shoes and, to the best of her ability, worked on her daughter's feet. Using zone theory to locate the appropriate area on the foot, she worked it to give her daughter some relief from the pain. It successfully dulled the pain until there was a doctor available! Later that day the girl's appendix was removed.

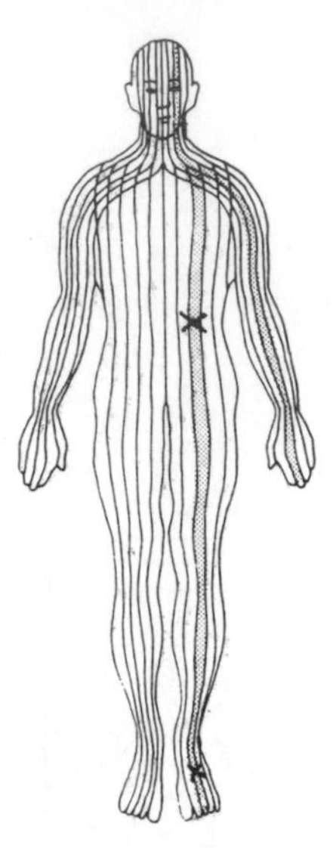

As a practice exercise, look at the illustration. Notice the spot marked "x" where, let's say, there's some pain or injury. By tracing along the appropriate zone down into the foot, you can find sensitivity there too. Since the basic principle of reflexology is that buildup will occur in that zone of the foot as a result of the stress or injury in spot "x", the zonal relationships provide guidelines for locating more pain more precisely. Using this information source in conjunction with the lateral zones on the feet (See pg. 6) permits the reflexologist to concentrate the effort on special target areas to relieve the trauma.

REFERRAL AREAS

An injured or affected part should never be worked on. This includes varicose veins, phlebitis, sprained ankle, or any limb or joint injury. Reflexology and zone theory allow us to select alternate parts of the body in the same zones and work them instead. This system is called "referral areas". Referral areas are different parts of the body that relate to each other through the zones. They are very valuable because of what they tell us about what's going on in the zones. They also provide excellent areas for self help homework, so that the client can amplify the reflexologist's efforts between treatments. When an area must be avoided entirely (due to an injury), the referral area is the alternative for working the zone.

Just how the limbs are related to each other through the zones is really quite simple. Each relationship is specialized. For example, compare your right arm and leg to the illustration. The arm is a reflection of the leg in zone terms. The hand corresponds to the foot, the wrist to the ankle, and so forth. If any part of the arm is injured, the corresponding part of the leg can be worked (and vice versa). Common problems such as phlebitis and varicose veins in the legs can be helped by working the same general areas of the arms.

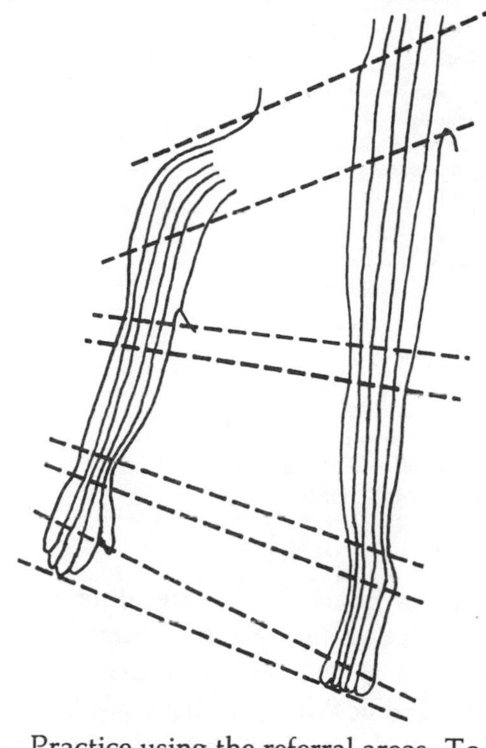

SHOULDER	—	HIP
UPPER ARM	—	THIGH
ELBOW	—	KNEE
FOREARM	—	CALF
WRIST	—	ANKLE
HAND	—	FOOT
FINGERS	—	TOES

Practice using the referral areas. To begin, set up the zones to get your bearings. Place your hands palms down on your knees. Number the zones starting with the thumb and big toe (Zone 1), the index finger and second toe (Zone 2), and so forth. Your picture may get a little distorted, though, because the arm and leg bend in "different" directions. When you placed your hands palms down, you rotated the radius bone of the arm. Now turn your hands over, palms up, and notice that the arm is straight but the zones no longer match. The thumb now seems to be in the same zone as the *little* toe. But it isn't. Use this perspective only to help you accurately find the part of the referral area to work.

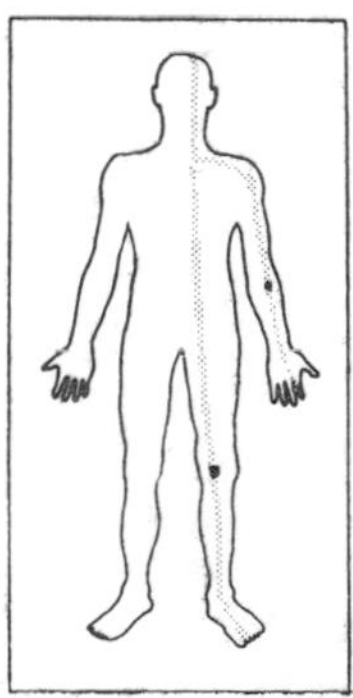

Look at the illustration. Where would you work for an injury to the inside of the left knee? Which zone is it in? Since it is in line with the second toe, we will call it "zone 2". Hold your left hand palm up. Start with the second finger and trace zone 2 up to the elbow. This would be your referral area for this particular knee injury. If you actually did encounter an injury here, you would probably find tenderness in the referral area of the elbow.

Case in Point:
A friend of ours who is a physical therapist became most interested in referral areas after we demonstrated to her a rather dramatic one on her own body. She had sustained a severe dogbite a few months before and the muscle had been damaged. She showed Kevin the evidence of the wound on her leg. He immediately "referred" to the corresponding part of her arm and began to probe around, looking for tenderness. He found it. There was a definite referral area on her arm that was surprisingly tender to the touch!

The same approach can be used to locate other referral areas. Identify which zone(s) an injury has occurred in and simply trace it to the referral area. Often the tenderness in the referral area will help you find it. With your hand palm up you can see that, contradictory as it may seem, the fleshy part of the forearm is the referral area for the fleshy part of the calf of the leg. The boney part of the forearm corresponds to the shin. The same holds true for the upper arm and thigh, with the front of the thigh corresponding to the tricep (back) of the arm.

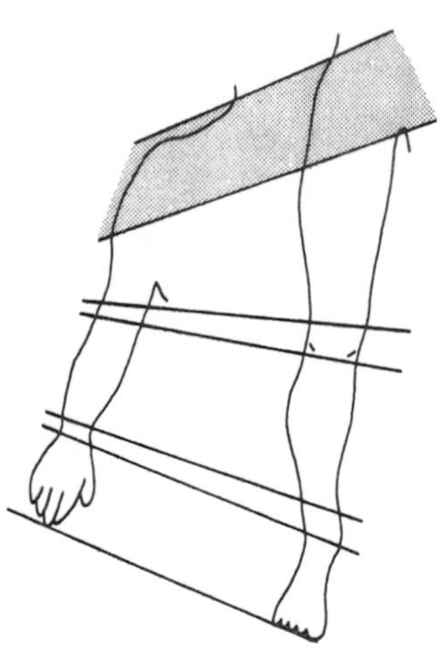

The importance of referral areas cannot be exaggerated. They can give insights into the problem areas by showing the relationships to the areas in the same zone(s) that may be at the root of a problem. Take a shoulder problem, for example. Because the shoulder lies in the same zone as the hip, a hip problem could be aggravating the shoulder. Referral areas point out just one more way the body operates as a whole.

The finger and thumb walking techniques (See pg. 23) can be adapted for use in working referral areas on the body. Often it is most efficient to walk all four fingers side by side through an area. When working a referral area on the knee or elbow, remember that the reflexes do pass through. Instead of trying to work the boney side (kneecap or elbow bone), find the corresponding area in the soft, fleshy crook of the joint.

WHY DOES REFLEXOLOGY WORK?

Although we know that zone theory and reflexology work, the actual mechanism involved, that is, why there are ten zones in the body arranged as they are, is not fully understood. It could be neurological, it could have to do with "energy pathways" not commonly considered as normal pathology, it could be circulatory — whatever the answer, further research and the continuing development of reflexology will help us find it. What we CAN talk about are the *results,* the observed effects of applied reflexology on the feet.

Perhaps the greatest ambition any reflexologist can have is to negate the effects of stress (and the resulting calcium buildup in the feet) for each and every client. For our purposes, we can think of stress as any influence impinging upon the body's ability to maintain homeostasis (equilibrium). So why does reflexology work? Let's take a closer look at what stress is all about.

STRESS — MORE THAN A FEELING

Stress and tension are no longer words associated only with the executive in the boardroom. The stewardess serving the passengers is under more stress than the pilot flying the plane. Each one of us, young or old, city or country dweller, lives with stress.

Imagine an incident of extreme stress: a threat of bodily harm. A primitive system, the "fight or flight" reaction, takes over. Instantly the body prepares to do battle or run. Hormones are released. The most notable, adrenalin, stimulates heart action and raises the blood pressure. Adrenalin also releases fuel in the form of glucose or stored blood sugar. More blood is sent to the muscles, the air passages become relaxed, and a sense of excitement is produced. Since other body functions such as digestion and excretion are not high priorities, adrenalin also causes vascular constriction which reduces the flow of blood to these areas. When the threat is over, blood flow returns to normal and the body returns to homeostasis.

The body uses adrenalin to cope with all kinds of stress. Obviously the stresses of every day life cannot be resolved with a weapon or a pair of track shoes, which often leaves the body keyed up and unable to return to homeostasis. If the body is subjected to regular doses of stress over an extended period of time (as most are), the effects are cumulative and it becomes more and more difficult to return to homeostasis. Here, research tells us, we have the root of 80 — 90% of all illness. The body simply cannot cope.

". . . the body is actually an aggregate of about 100 trillion cells organized into different functional structures, some of which are called organs. Each functional structure provides its share in the maintenance of homeostatic conditions in the extracellular fluid, which is often called the internal environment. As long as normal conditions are maintained in the internal environment, the cells of the body will continue to live and function properly. Thus, each cell benefits from homeostasis, and in turn each cell contributes its share toward the maintenance of the state. This reciprocal interplay provides continuous automaticity of the body until one or more functional systems lose their ability to contribute their share of function. When this happens, all cells of the body suffer."

Guyton, Arthur G.,
Basic Human Physiology, 1971, p.8

The cardio-vascular and digestive systems are obvious candidates for the ill effects of stress (i.e. high blood pressure, ulcers, indigestion, etc.). Stress may also be linked to infectious diseases. When the body is busy with the effects of residual stress, it cannot organize an effective defense against invading organisms. It becomes a vicious cycle. Stress is introduced and the body reacts. The problem remains unsolved and the residual tension and their effects remain.

What is the solution? The issue is not that we face stress but rather how to cope with it. How do we relieve the body of its stress and return it to homeostasis?

The reflexologist has the ability to reverse the effects of stress and to free the body to seek its homeostasis. Working the foot triggers a reflex action in a corresponding part of the body. This action is simply to relax the tension, reduce the vascular constriction and let the blood and nerve supply flow more freely. The body can then repair itself unimpeded by the effects of stress. Oxygen and nutrients make their way again to areas where they are needed. Repairs are effected. Improved circulation can prevent the stagnation that leads to disease. Like a swamp that has not been drained, poor circulation breeds a variety of problems.

If the blood pressure (the pressure at which the heart pumps blood into the major arteries) remains high, other problems ensue. One of the major problems is arteriosclerosis or hardening of the arteries. Increased pressure within the arteries causes several problems. The heart, brain or kidneys are prime target areas. The increased pressure forces materials into the walls of the arteries. These materials build up, coating the insides. Blood flow is reduced which signals a hormone in the kidney to be released and the pressure is further increased. A vicious cycle has been formed.

How are other organs affected? Reduced blood flow to organs can inhibit the oxygen and nutrients to the cells. Without oxygen the cell dies. Without the proper nutrients the cell fails to function efficiently. The glands and organs begin to malfunction and lose their balancing qualities. Depending on the *other* circumstances, they may overreact or underreact.

A good study of the body's balancing act is the pancreas. One of its jobs is to maintain the balance of glucose or blood sugar. It does this with its hormone, insulin, which gets the body cells to take up the glucose from the blood. Without insulin the glucose is not consumed or is stored improperly. It simply accumulates in the blood causing the dangerous condition called diabetes. If there is an excess of insulin produced the opposite effect is achieved. When the insulin removes glucose from the blood by increased combustion, the storage of glucose in the form of glycogen is increased at the expense of the blood. Low blood sugar or hypoglycemia (hypo = low) is the result. The balancing act has been upset. The glands and organs depend on an equilibrium. The blood circulation brings the needed elements.

Reflexology is aimed at restoring the lost balance. This is achieved through stimulating the reflexes in the feet to cause a relaxation in the corresponding body part. Improved circulation brings in the needed elements to repair and equalize the environment. The glands and organs in turn seek their equilibrium. The chain is completed.

To say it is simple would be deceptive. Reflexology acts on the body to release it to do its complex job of maintaining its many operations.

Blockages of the Zones

The foot, as a mirror image of the body, reflects any disturbances in the body's equilibrium in the form of blockages of the zones. Blockage is defined as a physical obstruction of a zone. Specific problems with a foot itself can also cause blockage. But by upsetting the homeostasis, stress can accumulate if not dealt with. Once this happens, blockage of one or more zones may occur in parts of the body where there is greatest vulnerability. It varies from person to person. What does NOT vary is the fact that stress, if not dealt with, will cause problems.

The feet act as self-tuners for the rest of the body. Movements of the feet stimulate the whole system. Unfortunately because of foot wear (and resulting lack of this stimulation), the feet are frustrated in their attempts to do their job. Reflexology retunes the system by applying alternating pressure on all parts of the feet. This has a corresponding effect on the zones throughout the body. A constant, direct pressure, however, has an analgesic effect on corresponding zones.

Over a long period of time, the use of constant, direct pressure can be harmful. It may deaden an area, causing it to become hypoactive (below normal). Circulation slows down. And then materials begin to deposit, which creates the blockages and further aggravates the problem. It may even have an adverse effect on the whole zone.

These symptomatic reflections of zonal imbalances manifest either as internal or external forms of blockage. Internal blockages are usually calcification or the pooling of lymph fluid. These are deposits below the surface of the skin. Since calcium is always present in the blood (approx. 1% of the body's calcium is constantly in circulation in the blood), it is readily available to be deposited. Tension and stress seem to cause this to happen. The feet are particularly prone to calcium buildup because they are at the bottom (gravity) of all the body's circulatory and waste removal systems. Also, they are under constant physical pressure. The deposits in the feet are commonly painful to the touch because they impinge on muscles and nerves. They can be quite large and very hard.

Lymph fluids in the body are transported by mechanical action (i.e., respiration, muscular) (See pg. 101). With an increase of tension in a zone, this lymph fluid can pool, causing problems for that zone. Pockets of lymph fluid in the feet can also become quite large.

External blockages occur on the surface of the skin. Corns and calluses are good examples of excess material formed in response to pressure, friction or repeated trauma. They block zones in much the same way as do internal blockages. For example, corns on the toes can be involved in neck and shoulder problems. Calluses on the ball of the foot can negatively influence many zones and organs, such as the lungs.

There are difficult questions. Does the problem of blockage of a zone by a corn or callus originate in the body and simply get reflected in the feet? For instance if there is a shoulder injury, would a compensating shift in posture and balance create new pressures on parts of the feet? It's really a "chicken or the egg" argument. In any event, corns and calluses are external blockages that affect the entire zones in which they occur.

It is clear that disorders of the feet can cause profound problems for the rest of the body. Bunions are frequently associated with neck and shoulder problems. Ingrown toenails put direct pressure on areas in the toes corresponding to the head region. The nails may become too thick or have unusual growths. Frequent headaches, eye/ear problems, strokes and old age senility are all potentially related to the toenails. It all points to the importance of proper nail care.

One final word. With specific foot problems such as corns, calluses, and ingrown nails, it may be necessary to seek the advice and care of a podiatrist. As a reflexologist, never hesitate to suggest this to your clients if the conditions warrant it.

The interplay between the body and its parts is a most beautiful, complex process. The relationship between the feet and the rest of the body obviously involves a number of factors. Blockages of the zones and general foot problems now appear to have far reaching and predictable impacts on total body health. In the following pages of this book we shall explore and illustrate exactly what it is that reflexologists do to intervene in these problems. This is information for anyone with hands and feet!

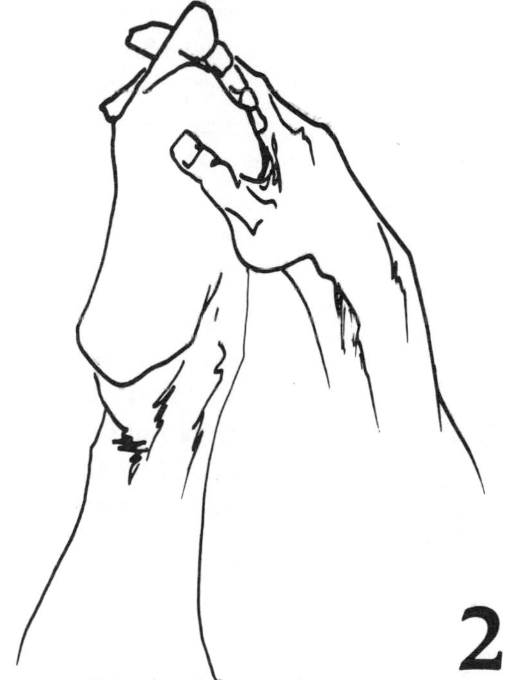

2

Techniques

Techniques

The techniques described in this chapter are designed to achieve two main goals: efficiency and effectiveness. In reflexology, efficiency is covering an area with the least amount of effort. Effectiveness is hitting the points, being dead-on-target in every area.

The three basic techniques are: the *thumb walking*, the *finger walking*, and the *thumb hook and back up*. Proper thumb motion covers large areas efficiently. *Finger walking* is a fine tuning technique for the tops and sides of the feet. The *hook and back up* pinpoints specific, hard to reach areas.

The three motions combined with leverage and proper holding of the foot form the basis of the techniques used in foot reflexology.

Holding the foot

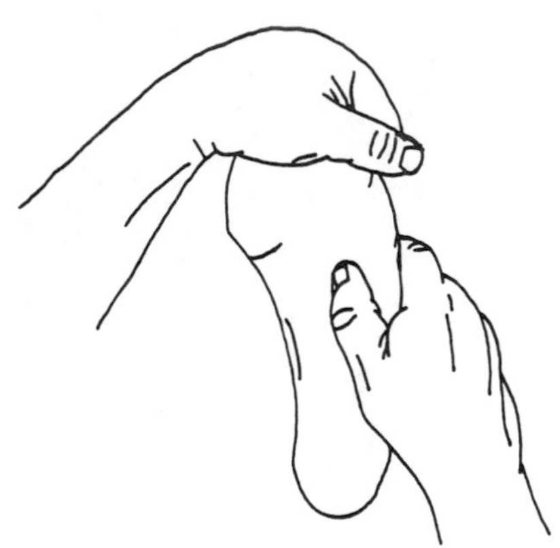

Holding the foot properly contributes to the overall effectiveness and efficiency of the three basic techniques. Proper holding facilitates walking with the thumb or fingers because it provides a stationary target and thins out the flesh so that the reflex points can be reached. The hand responsible for holding the foot in all of the techniques will hereinafter be called the "holding hand".

Detailed information on holding techniques is given with each technique section. In general, a stationary target is easier to hit than a moving one. So in reflexology, a stationary foot can be more effectively worked. One hand is then a "working" hand while the other is a "holding" hand. The working hand does the *thumb and finger walking* and the *thumb hook and back up* techniques. Each of the techniques has its own special holding problems. You must, then, become aware of how your holding hand is contributing to your effectiveness.

THE THUMB WALKING TECHNIQUE

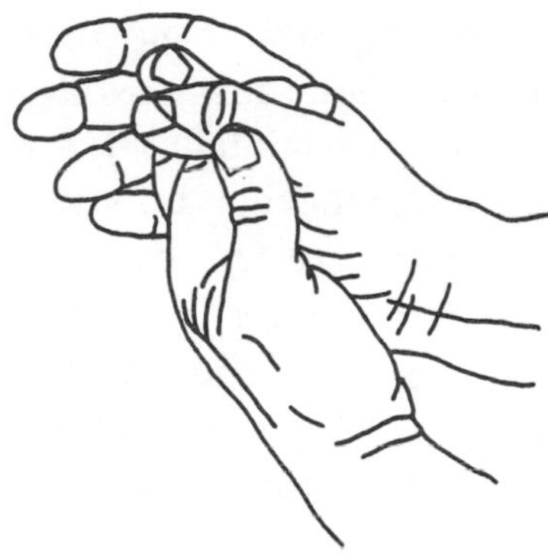

The *thumb walking* technique has a very simple basis: the bending of the first joint of the thumb. Try this exercise: hold the thumb below the first joint (as shown). This prevents the second joint from bending. Bend the first joint. Do it several times. Now try the other thumb.

While you're still holding, place the outside corner of the thumb on your leg. Bend the thumb a few times. At this point, do not worry about exerting pressure or about what your other fingers are doing.

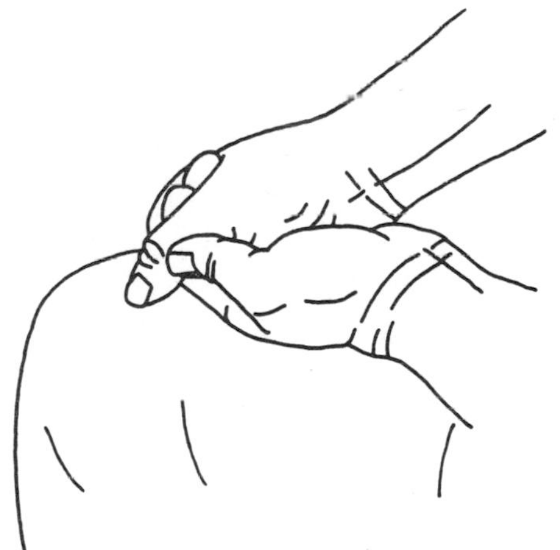

The next step is to get the thumb actually walking forward. Hold on to your thumb. Use the outside tip. Bend the thumb allowing it to rock a little from the thumb tip to the lower edge of the thumb nail. This is not a large range of motion; it is not meant to be.

Remove the holding hand. Try walking the thumb. Are you bending only the first joint? Do not push the thumb forward. Bending and unbending is the entire means by which you move forward.

It is at this point in our discussion of technique that an important aspect of efficiency arises. The fact is that actual strength in reflexology comes from the use of LEVERAGE. In the *thumb walking* technique, leverage is attained by the use of the four fingers in opposition to the thumb.

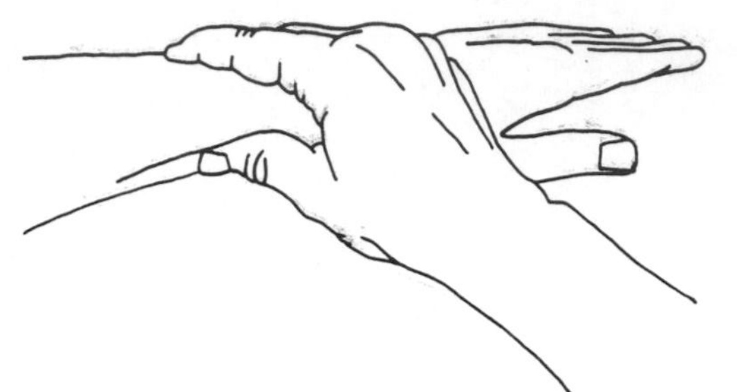

To practice using leverage, place the four fingers of the working hand on the opposite forearm (as shown). Keep the fingers and hand in the position shown. Lower the wrist of the working hand. You will be pulling and holding on with the four fingers while the thumb is pressed into the forearm. Maintain this position with the wrist lowered and allow the thumb to walk. Note the increased pressure now exerted by the thumb. The leverage provided by the fingers and the position of the wrist regulate the strength of the thumb. So the rule of leverage for thumb walking is: **Raise the wrist — lower the pressure. Lower the wrist — increase the pressure.**

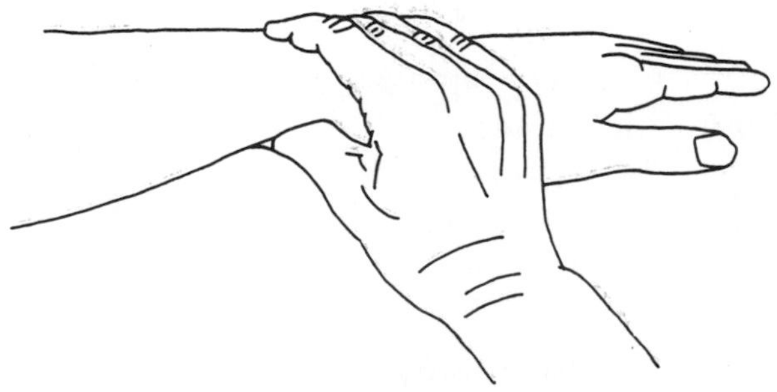

Refining the Thumb Walking Technique

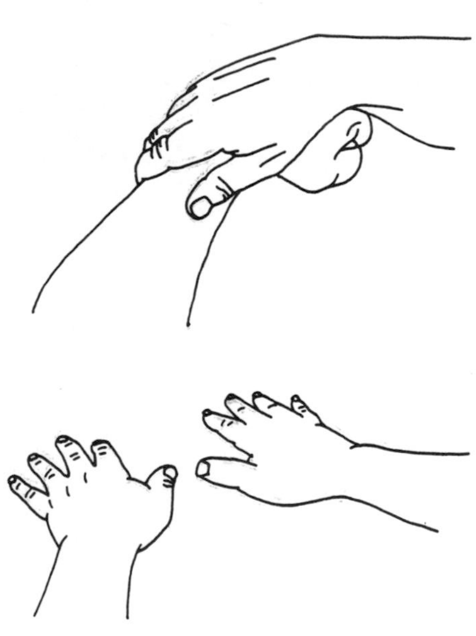

It is essential to walk the thumb with a constant, steady pressure. Practice on your forearm. Walk the thumb, taking smaller and smaller bites. Practice until you feel the steady pressure. **You should not feel an on-off-on-off pressure at each bend of the thumb.**

Finally, achieving good leverage means learning the proper *angle* of the thumb. Lay your hands down on a table or flat surface. Note how the thumb rests on the table. Walk it in this relaxed position. The outside edge now making contact with the table is the part of the thumb that should make contact with the foot. It can be described as the area from the lower outside edge of the nail to the tip of the thumb. By using this portion of the thumb correctly, you take best advantage of the leverage available from the four fingers.

APPLYING THE THUMB WALKING TO THE FEET

Now let's apply to the feet what we have learned. The *thumb walking* technique is most effective for covering the large areas on the bottom of the feet. There is quite a bit of flesh between your thumb and the reflex points. Therefore, the holding hand will be used for foot control, to thin this flesh out and to give the thumb a chance to work the necessary areas. In most instances this means holding the toes back with the holding hand.

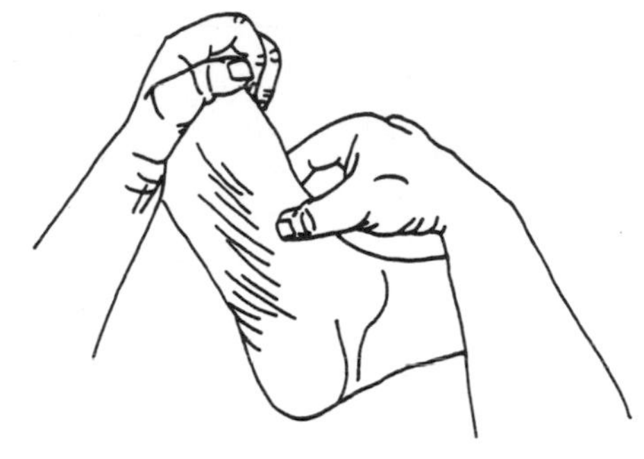

With your holding hand grasp the toes of a friend's foot. Hold them back (as shown). Feel for the tendon with your working hand. Avoid it for the moment. Now practice walking with the thumb on the bottom of the foot. Are you applying a constant, steady pressure? Are you walking on the corner of the thumb? Remember: the thumb ALWAYS moves forward, NEVER backwards or sideways.

While your thumb is walking on the bottom of the foot, notice what your leverage fingers are doing. They should be in a firm but natural position. If the thumb begins to walk away from this natural hand position, the hand is stretched out and leverage is lost. It is necessary to constantly re-position the fingers to maintain the essential leverage. Incidentally, the four fingers work as a unit and should be kept together. When the fingers are spread apart, some effectiveness is lost. If one or more fingers is lifted off the surface, even more leverage effectiveness is lost.

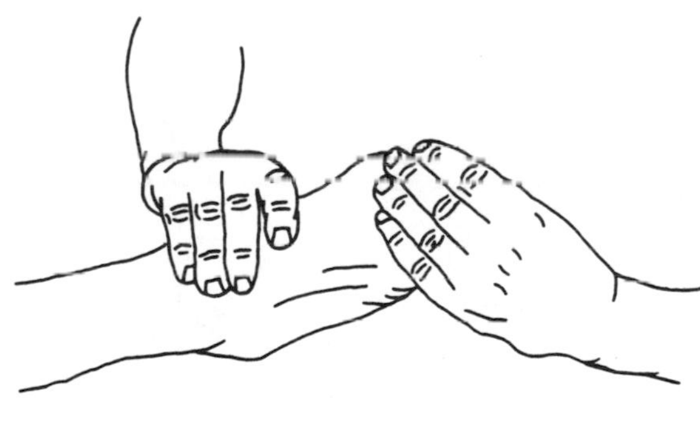

It will take practice to perfect your technique. Don't be discouraged. This is a whole new thing for your thumb to learn. Be patient and keep trying.

TROUBLE SHOOTING / SORE THUMBS / THE FINER POINTS OF LEVERAGE

If you have difficulty with your *thumb walking* technique, or if your use of leverage is inadequate, several problems will arise. You may not hit the point effectively. You may be rocking the thumb too far and hitting the foot with the thumb nail. And your thumbs may get sore.

Sore thumbs aren't necessarily a sign of poor technique because building strength in the thumb takes time. But sore thumbs may well point to weaknesses that can be easily corrected by reviewing the technique. Are you trying to press your thumb at each bite? If so, your thumb has every right to be sore! Test your thumb technique on your forearm or on someone else. Are you giving a feeling of on-off-on-off pressure? How much are you bending that first joint? If you're bending to the point that the nail hits the skin, back off a little. (See illus.)

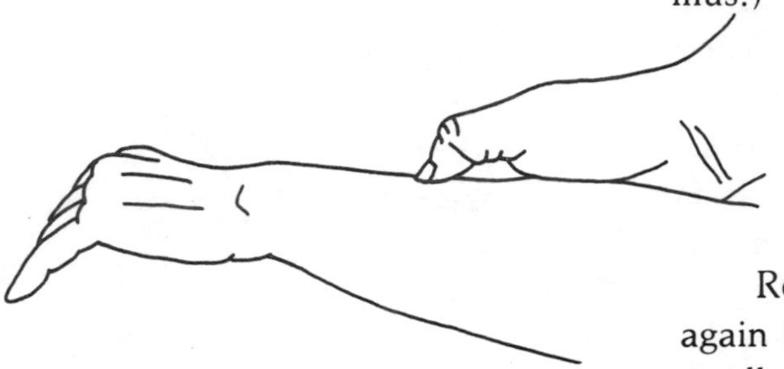

Rethink the thumb technique. Bend your thumb again from the first joint. Practice taking smaller and smaller bites until you can do it with constant, steady pressure. It cannot be over-emphasized. If you don't get it in one or two practice sessions, don't be discouraged. Keep trying. This is the basis for all walking techniques and must be mastered.

When you trouble shoot your technique think first of the cardinal rule: **constant, steady pressure combined with leverage allows you to effectively and efficiently hit the points.** If it seems to you that you *are* exerting this pressure but you still have problems, reevaluate your leverage.

Now let's review the finer points of leverage. First,

leverage is what your fingers do to help a walking thumb. When your thumb is walking, the fingers should be contoured to the shape of the foot. This permits you to use the strength of the whole finger. If the fingers are too curled, you use only the strength of each finger tip.

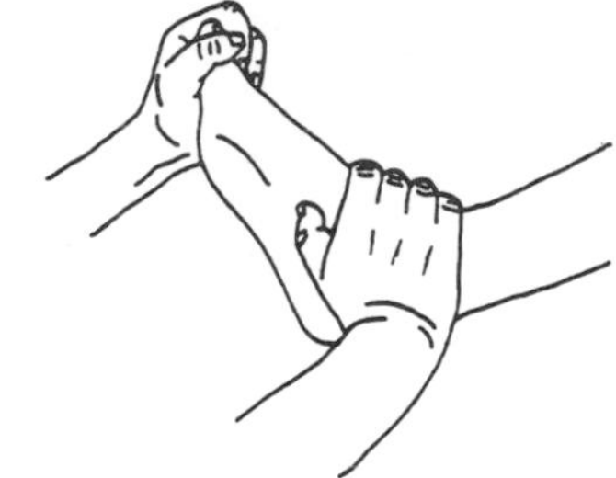

The four fingers should be kept together comfortably. When the fingers are spread out, some leverage is lost. The angle of the thumb also affects your leverage. Once again, using the corner of the thumb allows the most effective opposition to the fingers, thereby utilizing the natural strengths in the hand and fingers.

Each of the above considerations adds to the other to produce optimum leverage effectiveness. If you miss any one of the finer points, it detracts a bit from the most effective leverage.

THE FINGER WALKING TECHNIQUE

The *finger walking* technique has the same basis as the thumb: the bending of the first joint of the finger. Hold below the first joint (as shown). Bend the first joint.

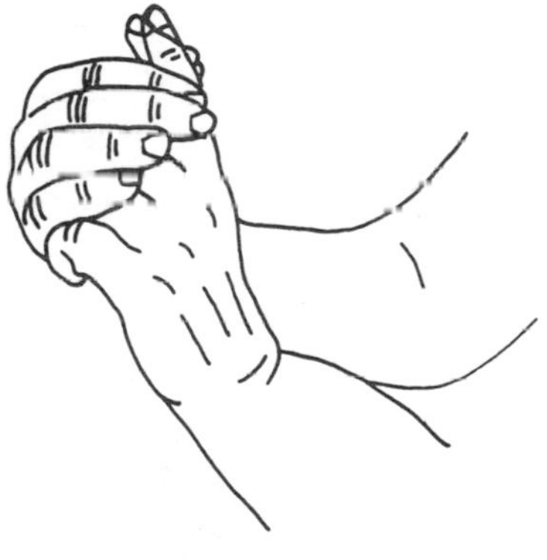

The top of the hand is a good practice ground for *finger walking*. Try bending from the first joint of the index finger as its tip rests on top of the hand. Use the edge of the finger. The walking motion is a slight rocking from the finger tip to the lower edge of the fingernail.

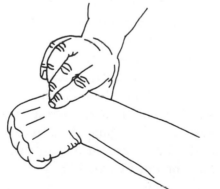

In the *finger walking* technique good leverage is attained by the use of the thumb in opposition to the fingers. To practice using leverage, place the four fingers of the working hand on the opposite forearm (as shown). Keep the fingers and hand in the position shown. Raise the wrist of the working hand. You should be pulling and holding on with the thumb. The fingers are pressed into the forearm. Maintain this position with the wrist raised and allow the index finger to walk. Note the increased pressure now exerted by the finger. The leverage provided by the thumb and the position of the wrist regulate the strength of the finger. So the rule of leverage for the *finger walking* technique is: **Raise the wrist — increase the pressure. Lower the wrist — lower the pressure.**

Practice this as you will all techniques. The goal is the same as with the thumb. Take smaller and smaller bites by exerting a constant, steady pressure. Avoid the on-off-on-off type of pressure. And remember, the finger always moves in a forward direction, never backwards or sideways.

Only one finger at a time does the actual walking. You need not use only the index finger. Any finger can effectively perform the technique.

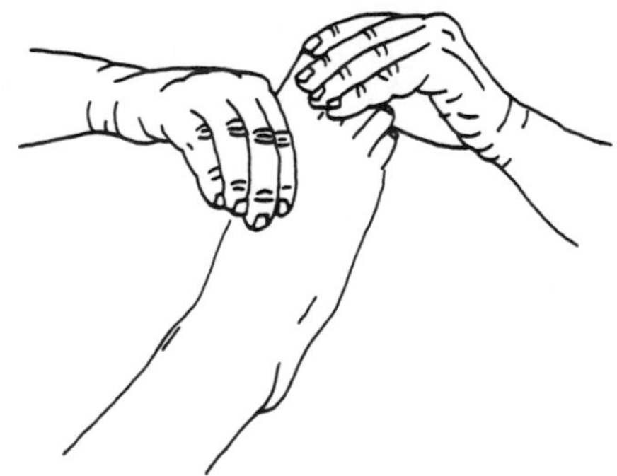

While one finger is walking, the other fingers contribute to the leverage by following along.

Problems can occur. Usually they involve difficulty in bending the first joint. Try to avoid the following: moving your hand excessively when walking the finger; digging the fingernail into the skin; allowing the walking finger to draw back rather than exerting a constant, forward pressure; merely rolling the walking finger from side to side. If you encounter any of these difficulties, review your technique by closely re-reading the description of the technique.

THE HOOK AND BACK UP TECHNIQUE/ PINPOINTING

The *hook and back up* technique is used to hit a particular point rather than to cover a large area. It is a relatively stationary technique.

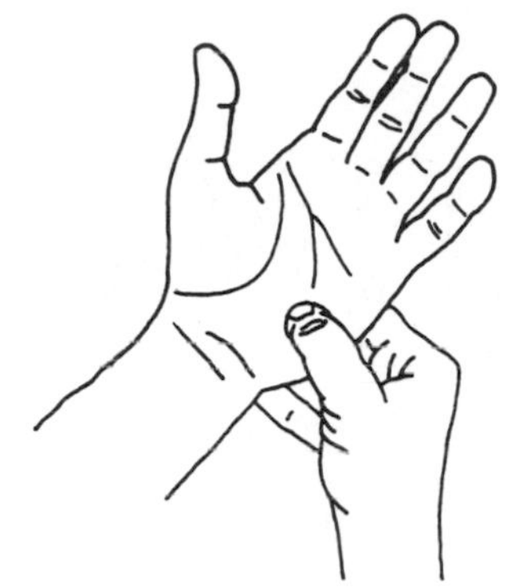

Rest your thumb on the palm of the other hand. Bring your fingers into contact with the top of the hand. Bend the first joint of the thumb, exerting pressure with the corner of the thumb just as you would with the *thumb walking* technique. Now pull back across the point with the thumb. This is the *hook and back up* technique.

As with all techniques leverage is extremely important in hitting these deeper points. Just as in the case of *thumb walking*, leverage is provided by the fingers and the position of the wrist (See pg. 24). Lower the wrist of the working hand and the pressure exerted by the thumb is increased. Maintain this position with the wrist lowered. Hook in with the thumb and pull back across the point.

A term that will be used to describe working the deep, specific points of the feet is "pinpointing". Since no walking is effective on such a small point, the *hook and back up* technique is used.

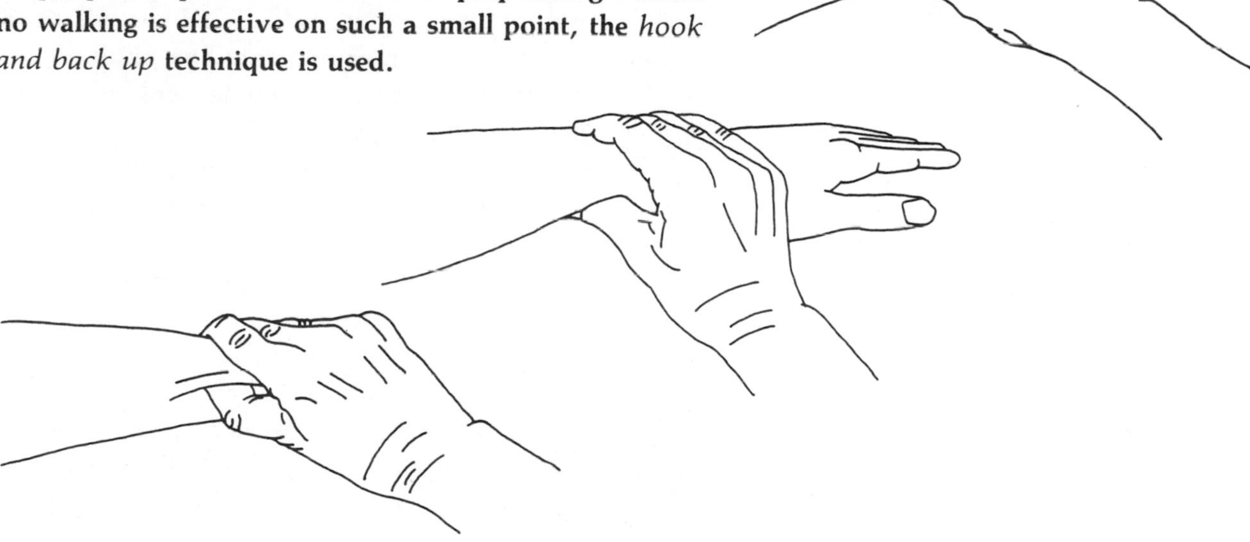

WORKING THE FEET

THE BIG TOE

pituitary
thyroid/parathyroid
7th cervical
top of the head

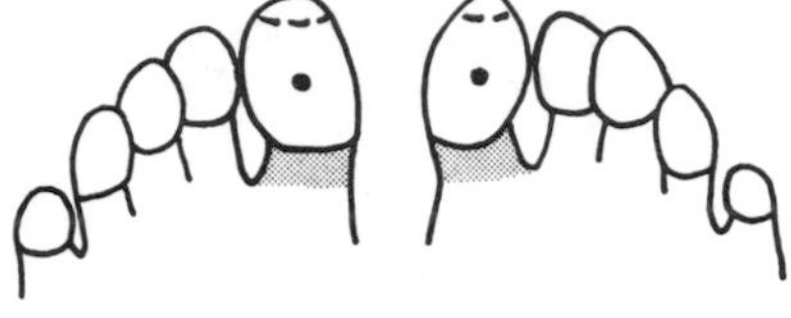

The big toe includes several important areas. Each toe represents half of the head area and contains all five zones. The head joins onto the body just as the toe joins the foot. The important connector between the toe and the foot then corresponds to the neck.

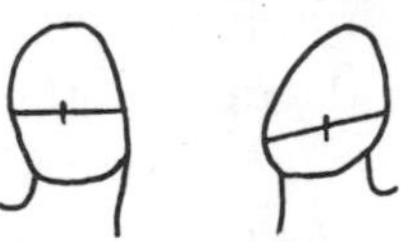

The **pituitary** is an exact pinpoint area. Locating the pituitary point requires measuring the big toe. Since big toes vary in shape and dimensions, it is important to use this measurement procedure. Look for the widest point on either side of the toe. Draw an imaginary line between these points (see Illus.). In some cases the widest point may be calloused. If the widest point is a callous use it for your measurement. The pituitary lies on the midpoint of this line. Some lines will be straight across, some will be slanted.

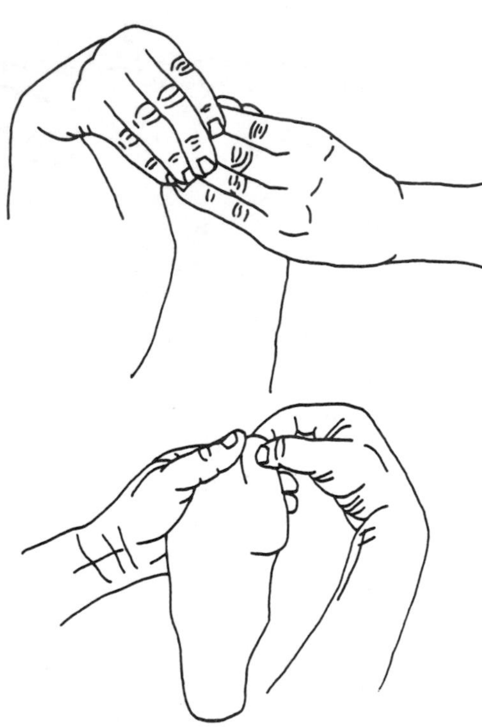

To work the point, you must support and protect your subject's big toe with the holding hand. This prevents excessive bending and pinching of the toe. Place the fingers of the working hand on those of the opposite hand. (See Illus.) Place the thumb just beyond the pituitary point. Use the *hook and back up* technique and be sure to use the corner of the thumb.

Leverage is very important here. Your right hand is the working hand on your subject's right big toe and so forth. This allows the fingers to provide the maximum leverage.

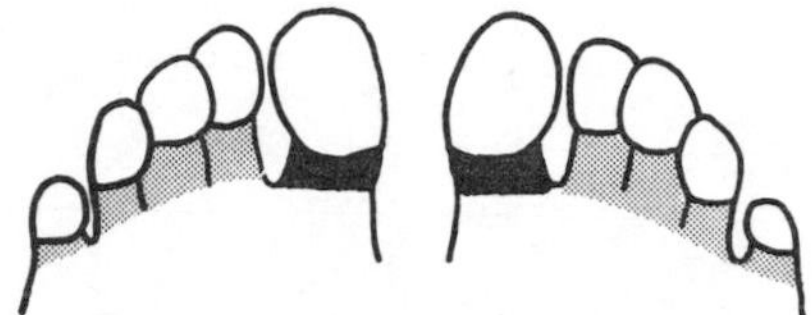

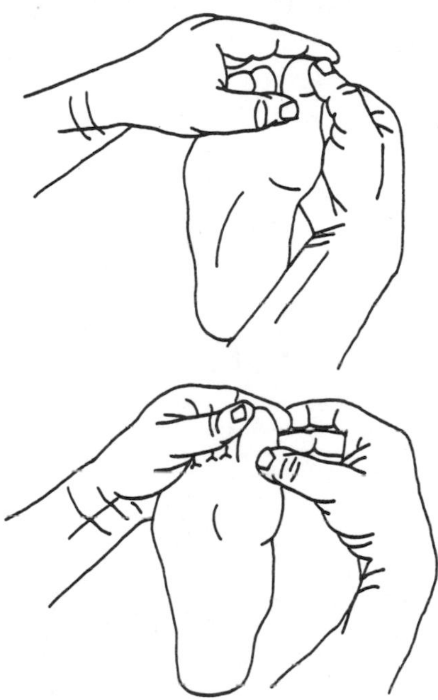

The **thyroid/parathyroid** are located above the base of the neck area on the toe. They are, therefore, located at the base of the big toe and of all the other toes. For the moment, we will discuss the technique for working this area on the big toe.

To work the thyroid/parathyroid area, support and protect the toe with the holding hand. Use the thumb to hold the toe to provide a stationary target. Place the fingers of the working hand on those of the holding hand (as shown). Walk across the area using the *thumb walking* technique. Make at least two passes, one high and one low. Several passes are necessary in order to cover the thyroid's wide area. Change hands and walk from the other direction. By working this and the 7th cervical area, you shall have covered the entire base of the big toe.

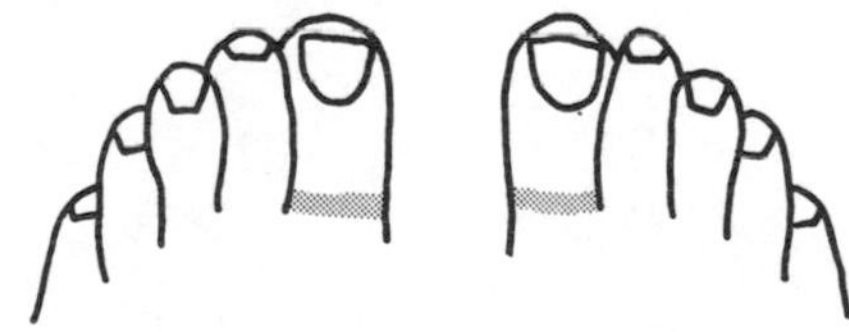

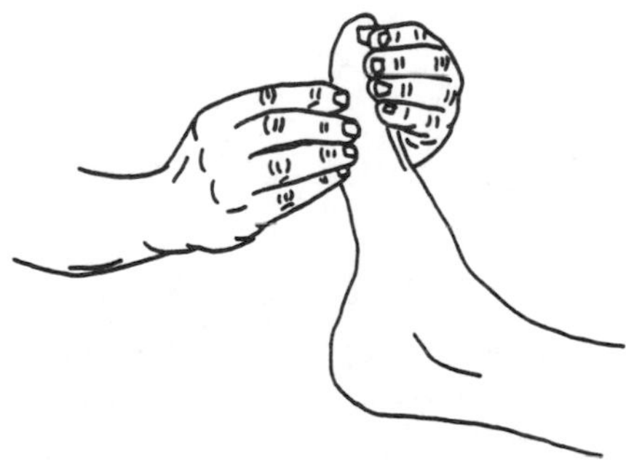

The **7th cervical** affects everything from the neck to the fingertips. Numbness in the fingers can often be traced to the 7th cervical.

To work the 7th cervical, start by anchoring the big toe with the fingertips and thumb. Place the thumb in a comfortable position on the bottom of the foot. Walk forward with the finger around the base of the top of the big toe. Angle the finger. Notice that you have walked around a groove at the base of the toe. An angled finger will fit into this area better than a thumb. (See Illus.)

THE TIPS OF THE TOES: TECHNIQUE VARIATION

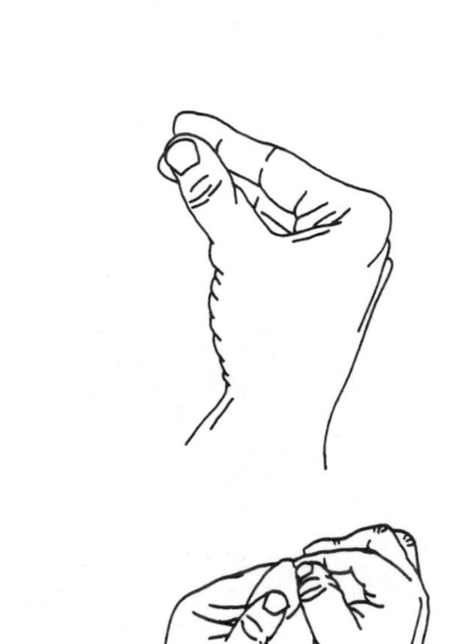

brain
top of the head

The tips of the toes represent the **top of the head.** Working this area can have special significance for head problems such as stroke, brain injury, and some eye and ear disorders. The big toe itself represents half of the head and is thus a focal point for this technique. The small toes can be worked in exactly the same way, however.

Anchor the big toe with the thumb and index finger of the holding hand. Either hand can be used. (See Illus.) Join the thumb and index finger of the working hand (as shown). Using the thumb as a support, roll the end of the index finger across a portion of the tip of the toe. The finger actually stays in place while you roll it from one side to the other exerting a downward pressure. Reposition the index finger and repeat. Cover the whole tip of the big toe in this manner. Repeat this procedure for the small toes. If you encounter sensitivity, take note. It is a guide to you for locating areas that will need special attention.

THE SMALL TOES: THUMB WALKING

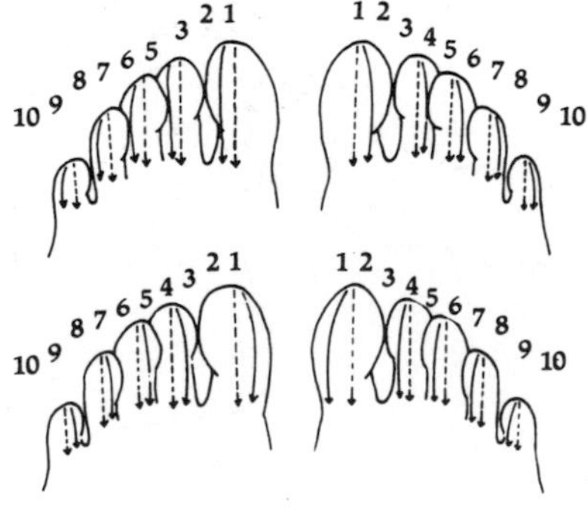

head/sinus
neck/thyroid

The small toes represent a breakdown of the big toe. They are in zones 2, 3, 4 and 5 respectively. The small toes are the fine tuning of the big toe.

The goal of this technique is to walk the thumb down the center and two sidepaths of each toe. There is a natural way that the thumb fits against the toes.

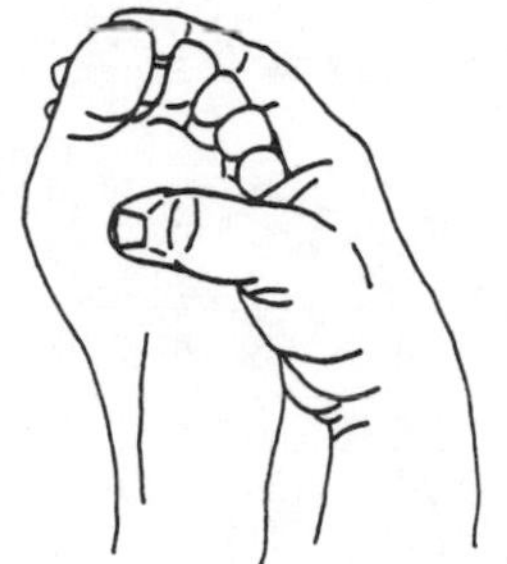

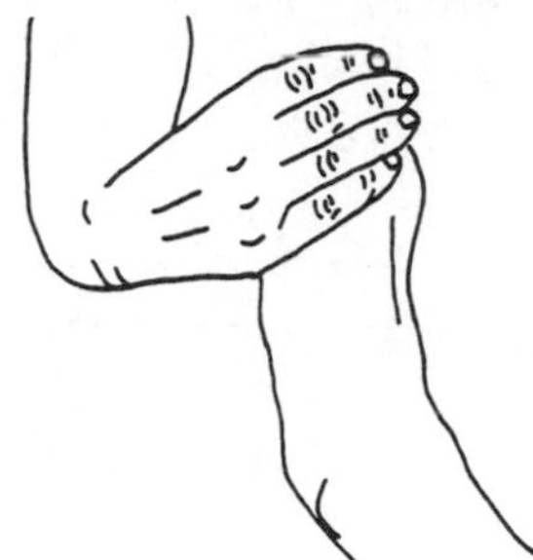

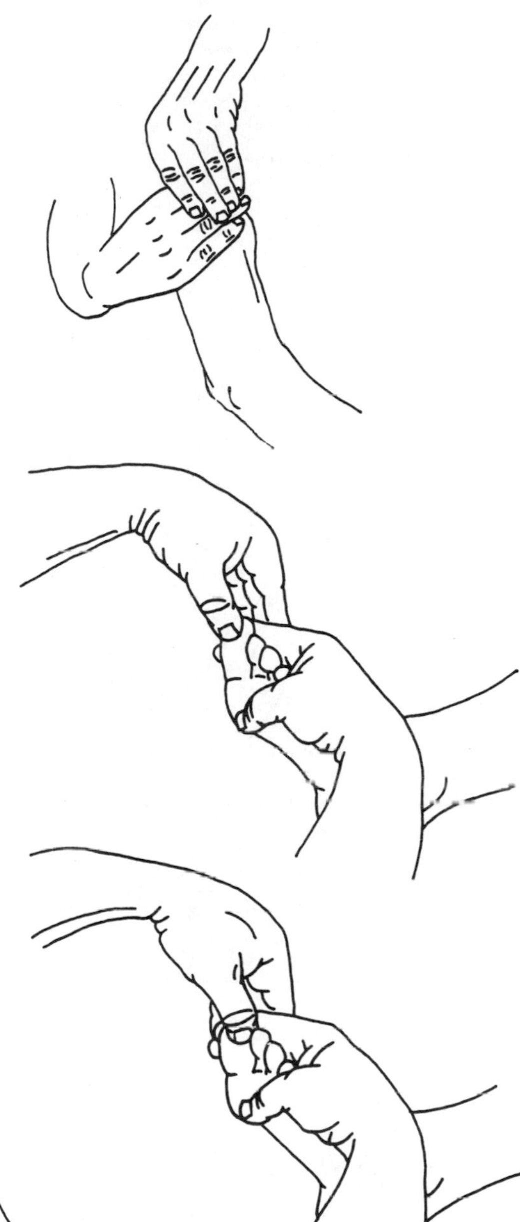

Begin by supporting and protecting the toes of your subject's left foot with the holding hand. The toes are flexible and would be difficult to work if not supported. Also they can be pinched easily which can be painful.

Bring your holding hand up to the tops of the toes, perhaps a little above. This will act as a backstop for leverage, comfort and control. Place the fingers of the working hand on the backstop fingers. (See Illus.) Starting at the top of the toe, walk with the thumb down pathway one. Even though the toes are small, they have many important areas. Cover them smoothly and thoroughly by using small bites. Remember to use the corner of the thumb. As you walk down pathway 2, you will notice that working the side of the toe is more difficult. Continue walking down the remaining pathways, but remember that the backstop hand follows the working hand curling around the toe to control it as the thumb walks down it. Work through the other toes in this manner. The important role the backstop hand plays will become clearer and clearer. After completing pathway 10, go right on.

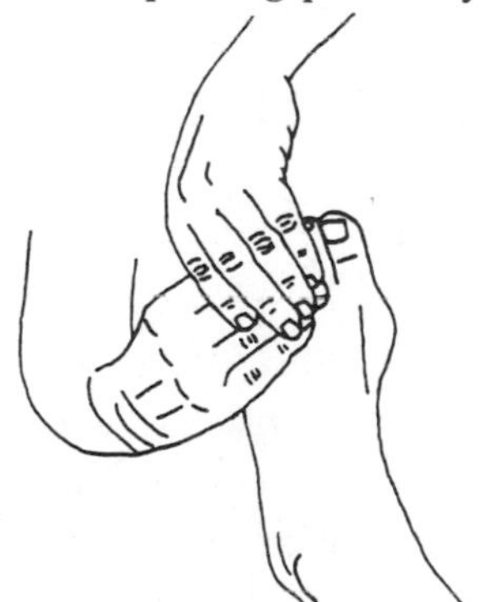

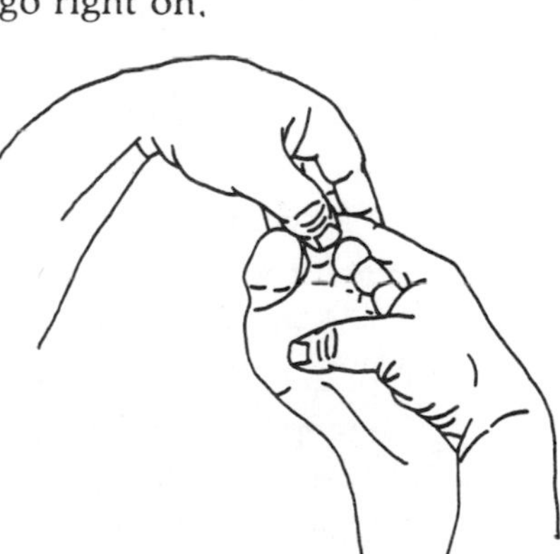

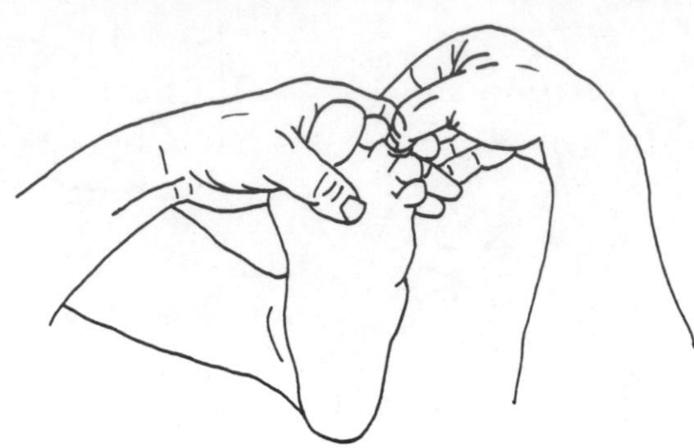

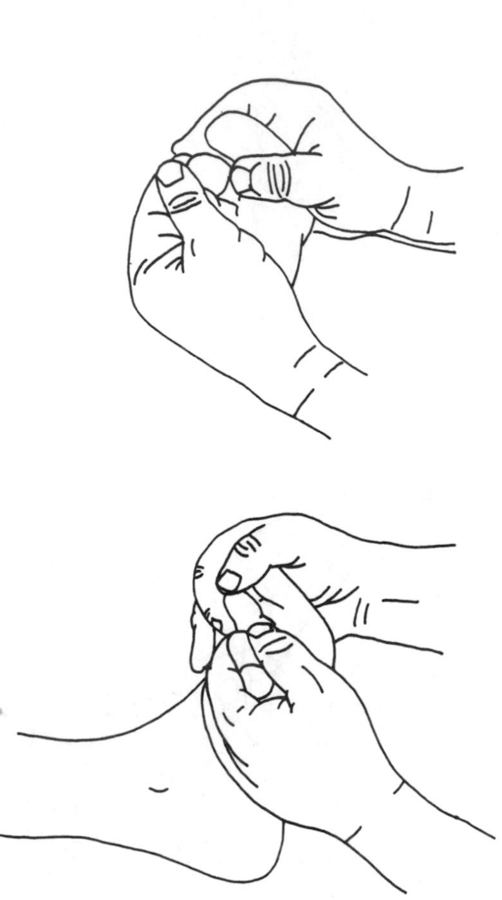

You are still working on the right foot. Change hands and follow the same method to walk down the bottoms of the toes. Remember to curl the holding fingers to control the toes. Follow the same procedure for working the small toes of the left foot.

To finish working the bottoms and sidepaths, walk *up* them the same way you walked *down* them. Use the thumb to walk from the base of each toe up each sidepath to the top of the toe. Then walk up the bottom of each toe from the base to the top. Change hands and work the other sidepaths and bottoms again (as shown). This part of the technique is beneficial for various problems in the head and neck area, particularly those in the neck muscles which are the prime candidates for storing tension and stress.

Note: This technique may not be possible with short or tightly curled toes. The sidepaths, however, can usually be covered on any toe, no matter how curled.

THE SMALL TOES: FINGER WALKING

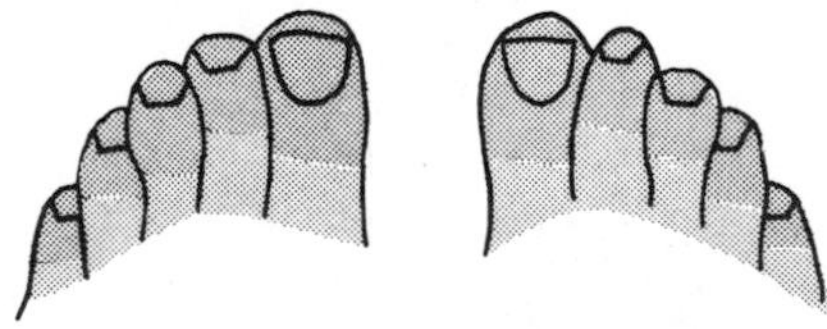

To complete the coverage of the small toes, the tops of each toe must be worked. The sidepaths and tops of the small toes are worked using the *finger walking* technique. If your subject complains of shoulder problems, it may be helpful to walk down into the lung area on the top of the foot as you work from the tops of each toe.

Use the thumb of the holding hand as a brace on the toe you work. Starting at the top of the toe walk the finger down the top sidepath and top center of each toe. Switch hands and cover the other top sidepaths.

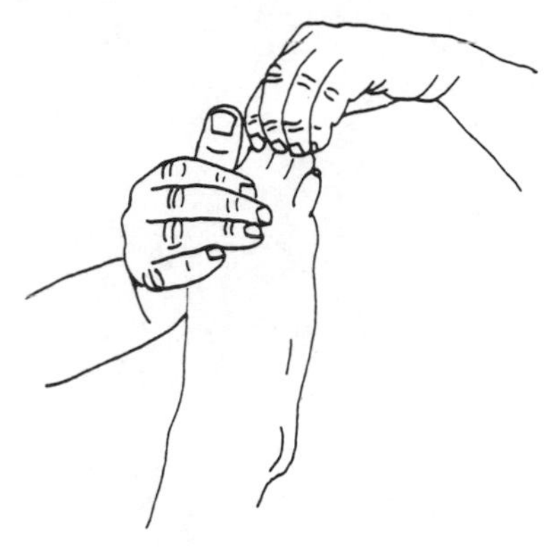

This technique will help you explore a variety of problems in the head-neck region. These include lymph, shoulder and tension. Be careful when using this technique not to stretch or hurt the sensitive skin between the toes.

THE RIDGE ALONG THE BASE OF THE TOES: THUMB WALKING

eye/ear

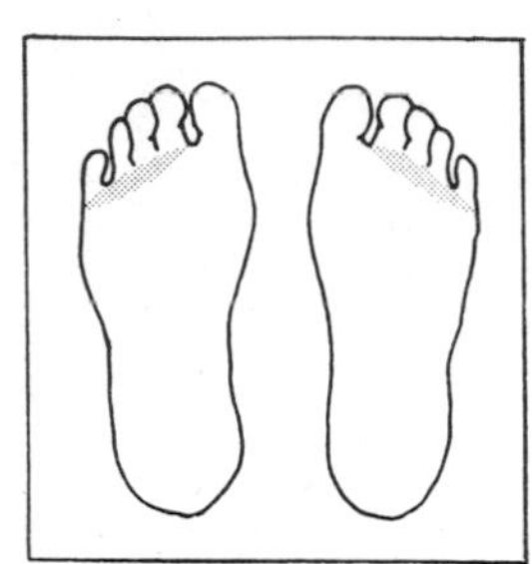

The object of this technique is to walk with the thumb along the ridge at the base of the toes. To maximize effectiveness, the flesh in this area must be thinned out.

With the holding hand pull the pad of the foot down to thin out this flesh (as shown). This opens the area up. Do not squeeze the foot because that would put more flesh between you and those reflexes. Do not hold the toes back either, for that would tighten the skin, making it even more difficult to work the area. Using the thumb, walk along the top of this ridge. Exert the pressure downward (toward the heel) along the top of the ridge. Do not walk against the toes or you will miss the reflexes.

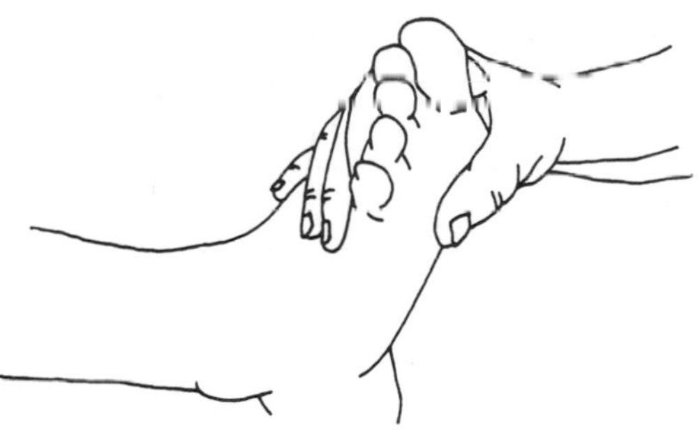

Change hands and walk across the ridge from the opposite direction. Walking from both directions insures hitting all points.

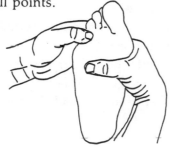

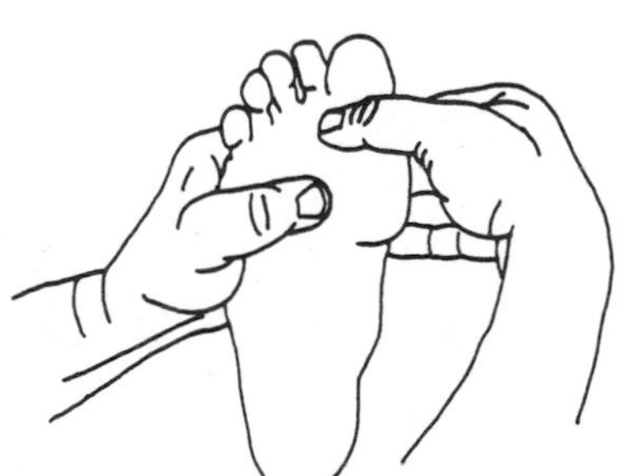

On the feet the eye and the ear areas overlap. Anatomically the inner ear is behind the eye. So on the foot the inner ear area is on the ridge between the third and fourth toes (as shown).

Note: In general the foot follows a logical pattern relating the anatomy of the body to areas on the feet. The location of the eye/ear area seems to be an exception. Even though the reflexes of the eyes and ears are probably located in the toes themselves, it has been found helpful to work the ridge at the base of the toes for eye/ear problems.

SOLAR PLEXUS/DIAPHRAGM AREA ON THE BOTTOM OF THE FOOT: THUMB WALKING

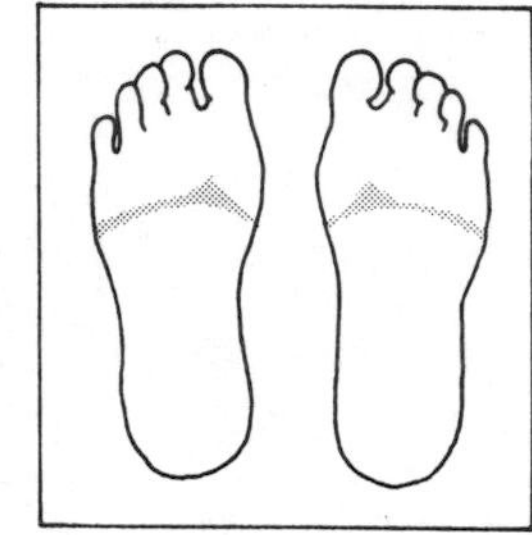

If one had to choose only one area on the foot to work, it would have to be this one. This reflex area is the body's midbrain, a nerve network with connections to all parts of the trunk and limbs. This is the primary target area for releasing tension and relaxing your subject (See page 15).

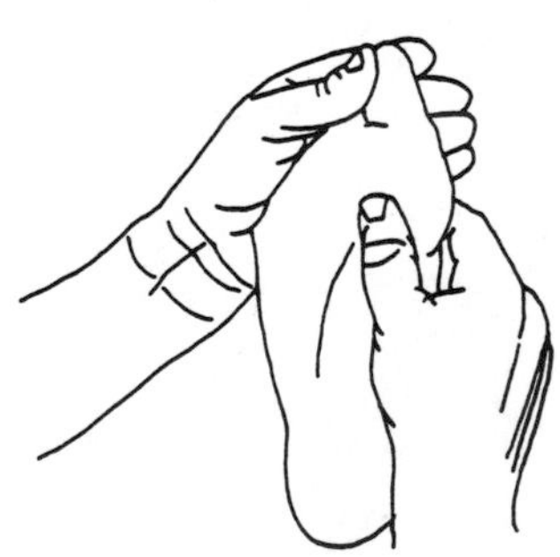

The thumb walking technique is used to work the area. On the right foot, hold the toes back with the left hand. Place the fingers of the working hand on top of the foot for leverage. Walk through the area with the thumb. Try it from several directions. Pay particular attention to the trough below the ball of the foot in line with the big toe. (See Illus.) Frequently, your subject will have stored a large amount of tension in this area. It is also associated with the hiatal hernia, a hernia of the wall of the diaphragm. This area on the left foot is usually more tender because the hernia is prone to occur more on the left side of the diaphragm. To work the left foot, reverse hands and repeat the procedure.

INTRODUCTION TO THE LUNG AREA

Reflexes pass through the foot. What this means is that the reflex areas listed as being on top of the foot can be worked from the bottom too. This does not mean that there is a "top of the lung" or a "bottom of the lung" area on the foot. Frequently it will prove easier to work these areas on the top of the foot because there is little flesh to inhibit your hitting the points.

LUNG AREA ON THE BOTTOM OF THE FOOT: THUMB WALKING

chest
lung
breast
shoulder

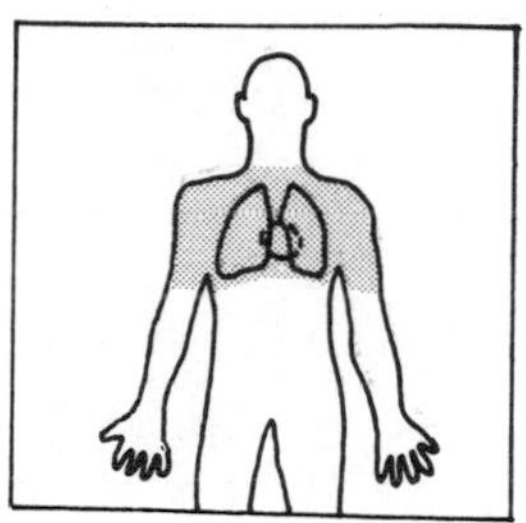

The picture of the body at the right is flat. But your body is three-dimensional. Imagine for a moment that this section is isolated from the rest of the body. On the front of it would be the shoulder, chest and breast. On the back are the shoulder, shoulder blades and the area in between. Sandwiched between are the lungs and heart. When you work the lung area on the bottom of the foot you touch all of these areas. The whole area extends from the base of the toes through the ball of the foot (See Illus.).

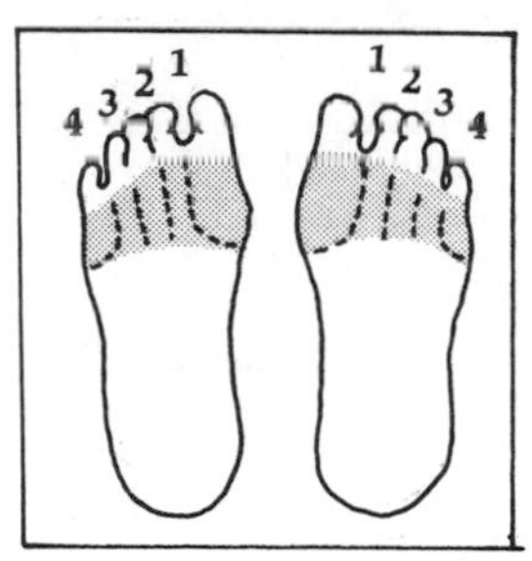

To work the lung area on the bottom of the right foot, hold the toes back with the left hand. This permits you to walk up the four troughs between the toes on the ball of the foot. Use the thumb to walk around the curved portion and up trough 1. (See Illus.) The starting point for this is actually the diaphragm/solar plexus. Do not worry about working both sides of the trough. Use the same thumb to walk up trough 2. Change hands (the thumb is more efficient if not stretched too far). Hold the toes back with the right hand. Walk up trough 3 with the thumb of the left hand. Use the same hand to

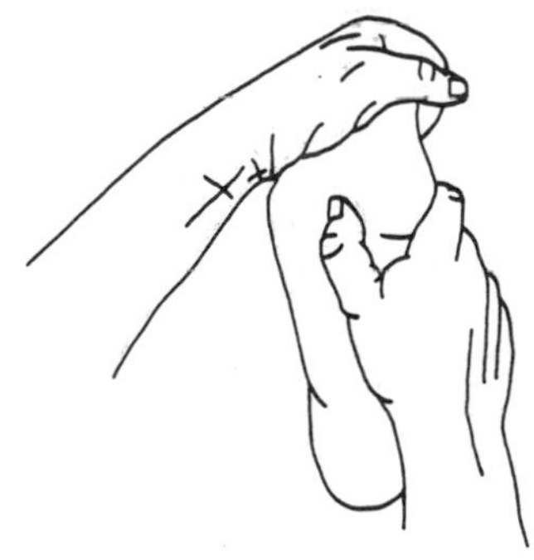

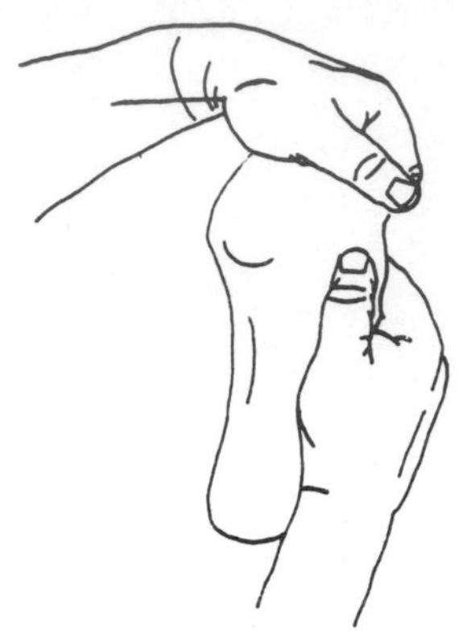

walk around the curve and up trough 4. This is the shoulder area.

To work the left foot, follow the same procedure. The right hand is now the holding hand. When walking through trough 1 on the left foot, one problem that may show up is a hiatal hernia. This is a ballooning of the esophagus through a weakened wall of the diaphragm. In this case, both feet will be tender in trough 1, but the left foot will be more sensitive.

LUNG AREA AND BELOW ON THE TOP OF THE FOOT: FINGER WALKING

chest/breast
lung
shoulder

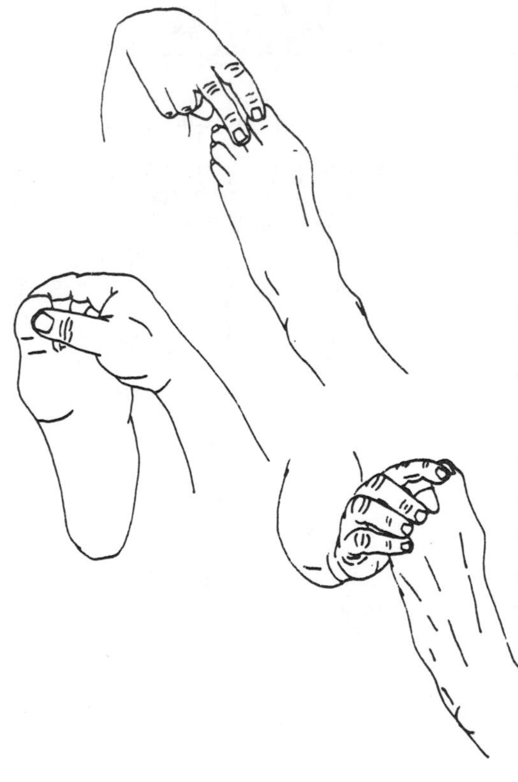

The object here is to work both sides of each of the our troughs on the top of each foot. These troughs are deep, so part of this technique involves exposing them through proper foot holding.

Refer to the illustrations . Beginning with the left foot, use the right hand as the holding hand. The index finger of the left hand does the walking. There are three important parts to this technique:

(1) To widen the troughs and make them easier to see and work, spread the toes apart. To do this, place two fingers of the holding hand (as shown) for stability. The thumb does the spreading.

(2) To open the area while providing a stationary object to work, push on the ball of the foot with the flat of the thumb of the working hand. Experiment pushing the thumb on the ball of the foot and watch how it exposes the troughs on top of the foot.

(3) With the index finger of the working hand, walk down trough 1 to the waistline. The left hand finger will do best on the left side of the troughs (your left). Use the index finger of the right hand for the rightside of the troughs. Using the correct finger ensures that optimum leverage will be attained.

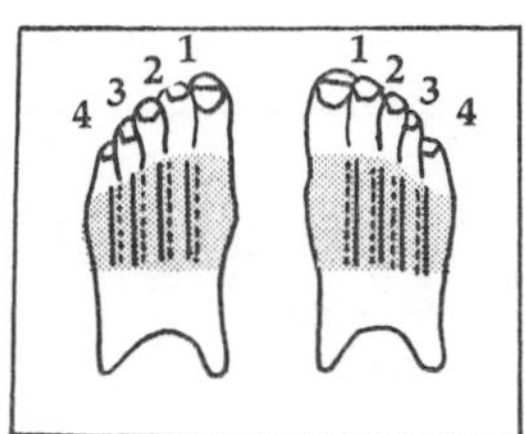

Work the rest of the troughs in the same manner. When you work the right side of the troughs, the left hand is the holding hand. The *finger walking* is especially critical in this technique. Any extra bending or unbending motion can cause nail marks or dragging of the tender skin on top of the foot.

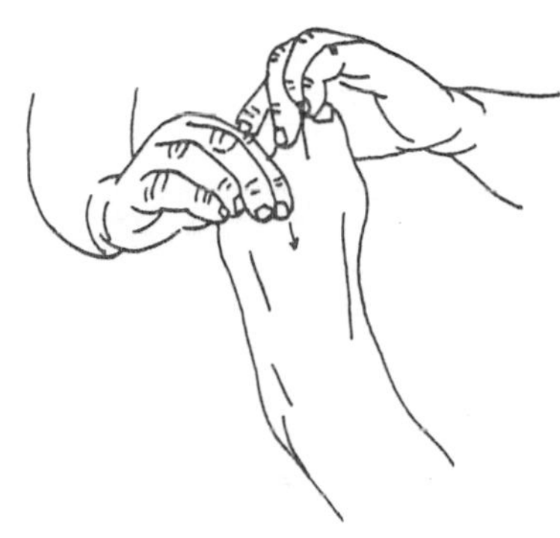

The walking motion must always be forward with a constant, steady pressure. The temptation is to hit the point by drawing back across it. This would cause pain or irritation. It is not a good way to hit the points. Rocking the finger too far with on-off-on-off pressure will leave a trail of fingernail marks on the foot. This is unnecessary.

The walking finger should be angled slightly. In addition to opening up the area, pushing up firmly with the thumb on the ball of the foot provides leverage for the walking finger.

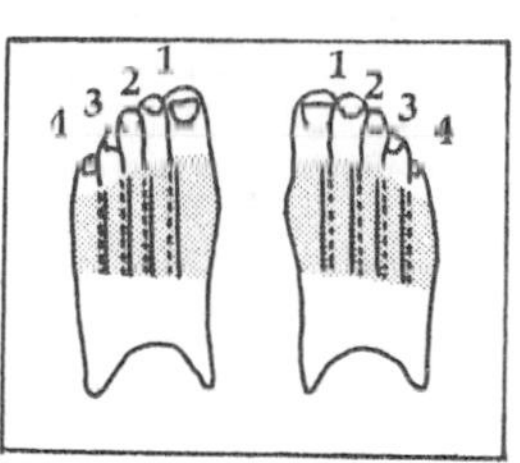

Wide feet can be difficult in this technique. It may be too difficult to stretch the hand around the toes to walk down the troughs. Try walking down one side of the trough. Then change your angle and walk down the other side. Do the first two troughs this way.

The *finger walking* technique for the top of the foot takes practice. Spreading the toes, pushing with the thumb on the ball of the foot, and walking with the finger are all equally important to a successful technique. When done properly, the technique is comfortable *and* effective.

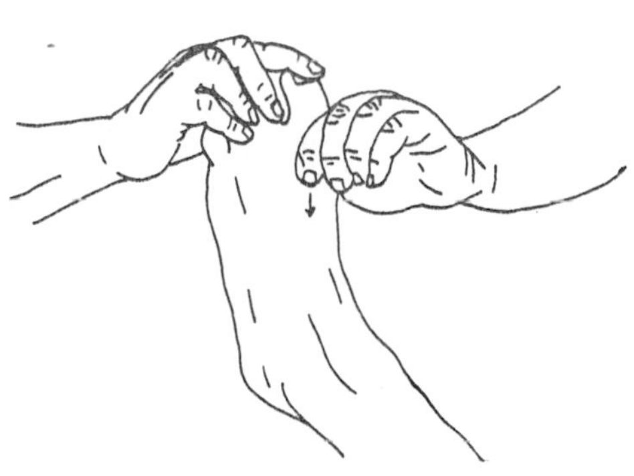

WAISTLINE AREA AND ABOVE ON THE BOTTOM OF THE FOOT: THUMB WALKING

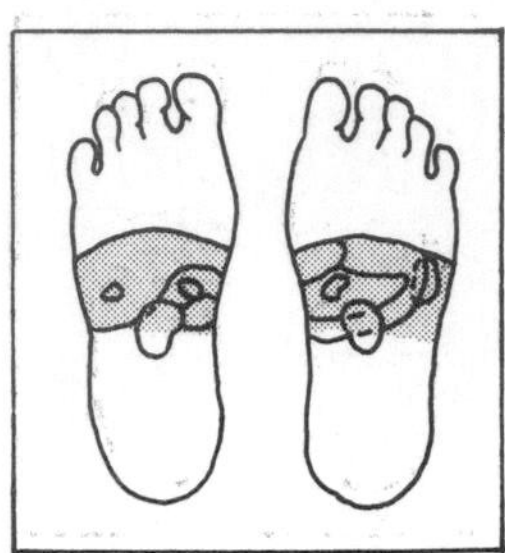

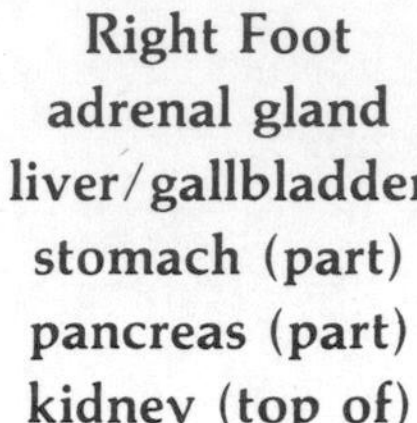

Right Foot	Left Foot
adrenal gland	adrenal gland
liver/gallbladder	spleen
stomach (part)	stomach
pancreas (part)	pancreas
kidney (top of)	kidney (top of)

As you can see from the above list, many vital organs are represented in this section of the foot. The *thumb walking* technique is used to work all of these reflexes in a very systematic way. For maximum effectiveness it is necessary to be conscious of the specific organs' reflex locations.

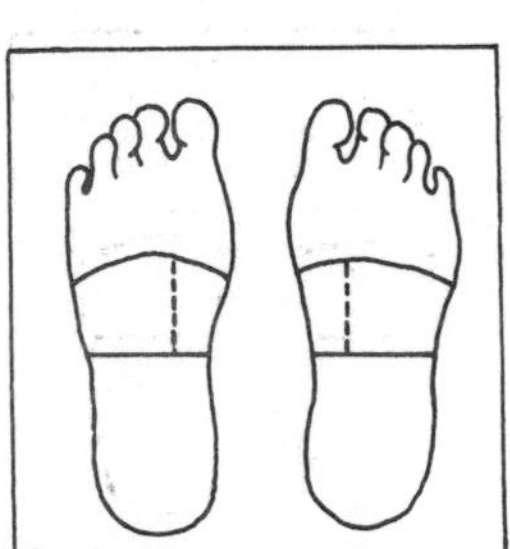

The region is bounded by the diaphragm and the waistline (See Illus.). On the foot the diaphragm is the area defined by the lower border of the ball of the foot. The waistline is an imaginary line drawn across the foot from the fifth metatarsal, which is the protruding bone midway down the outside of the foot. Find this bone on your own foot. Then draw a line from the high spot on this bone straight across the foot. This is your waistline.

Another locator is the tendon. It assists you in locating the adrenal glands and kidney areas. In the body the adrenal glands sit on top of the kidney. Both kidneys, however, are tilted. This causes the adrenals to lie on the inside of the tendon, and the kidney on the outside.

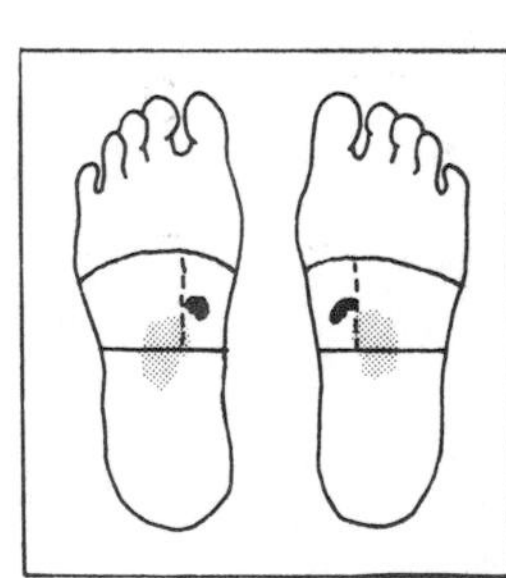

Look at your foot once again. Flex the toes. Notice that when you pull the toes back a rather thick tendon protrudes, running from the big toe back to the heel. If you have a thick foot, you may have to feel for it. The adrenal glands' reflex areas lie on the inside of this tendon halfway up the waistline to the diaphragm. All of the other vital organs can be located within the waistline-diaphragm-adrenal boundary.

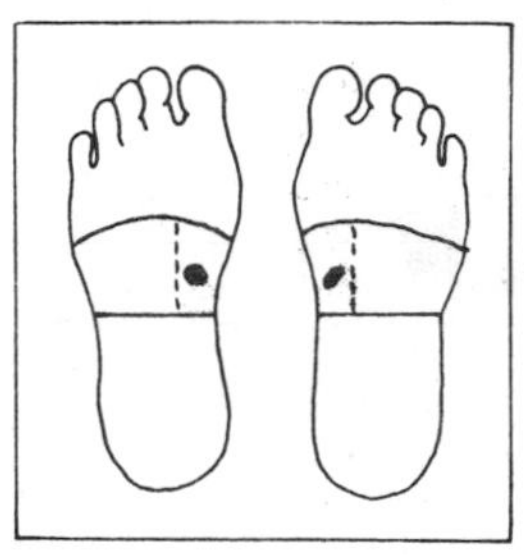

The pancreas fits below the adrenal gland with a slight upward slant. The majority of the pancreas area is on the left foot, but remember to work the small portion of it on the right foot.

The liver/gallbladder is a rather large area under the diaphragm line. It extends from the outside of the right foot all the way across to the left foot. The gallbladder is located on the right foot but may vary a bit in location.

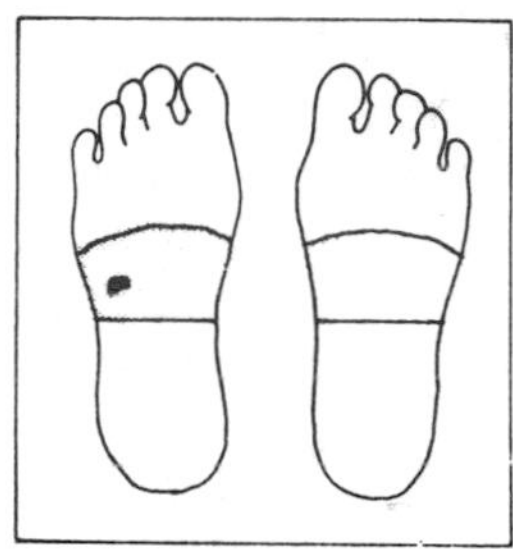

The spleen is positioned under the diaphragm line on the left foot. Much smaller than the liver, it is located at the tail end of the pancreas.

The stomach lies mostly on the left foot overlapping several areas. The duodenum, the prime candidate for ulceration, lies on the right foot just to the outside edge of the pancreas.

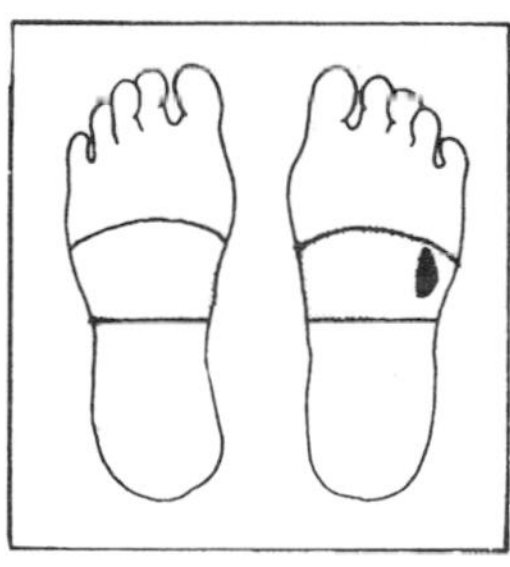

Slightly above the waistline on both feet are parts of the kidney and large colon. The kidneys are positioned along the waistline with the left kidney slightly higher. When working this area on the outside of the tendon, you encounter the top half of each kidney.

Parts of the large intestine run through this area. Working the large intestine, however, is discussed in the section on the *waistline and below* (page 44).

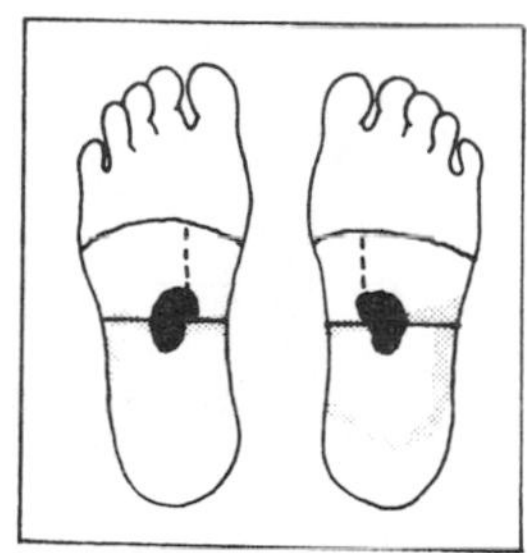

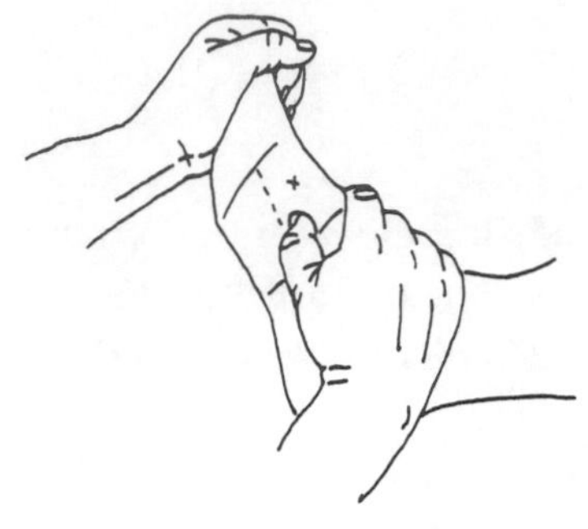

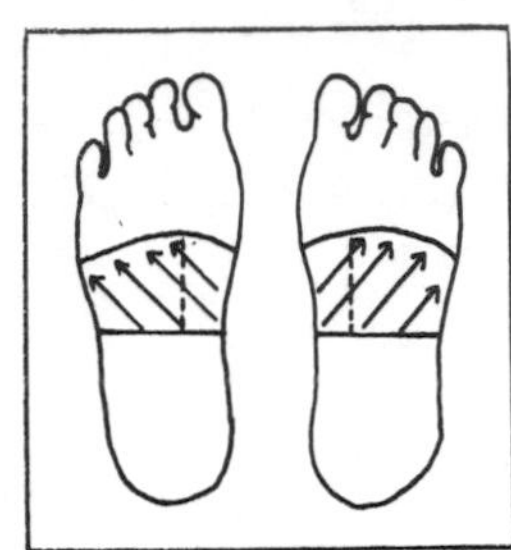

When working on the feet, there is a suggested order to working these reflex areas. On the right foot use the left hand to hold. Walk in to pinpoint the pancreas. Starting at the waistline on the inside of the foot tendon, walk with the thumb along the tendon until you locate the adrenal glands area. Then work diagonally across this area, letting up on the tendon as needed. Change hands and walk the other thumb diagonally through the area. Make several passes. But set up some kind of pattern for yourself so that you do not miss even the smallest part of the area. You should be working the entire waistline to diaphragm area at this point. Cover it thoroughly.

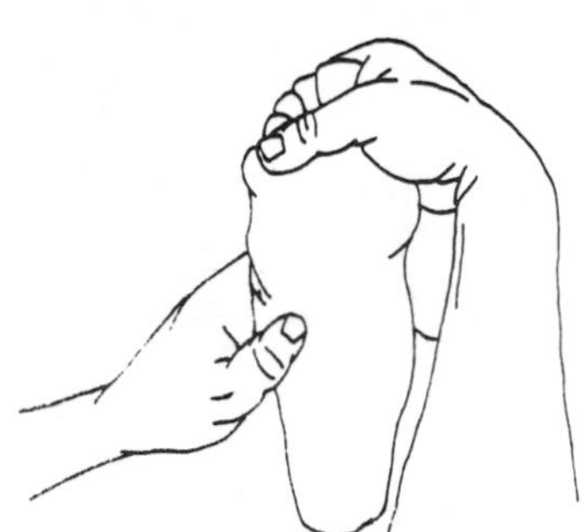

Repeat the procedure for the left foot.

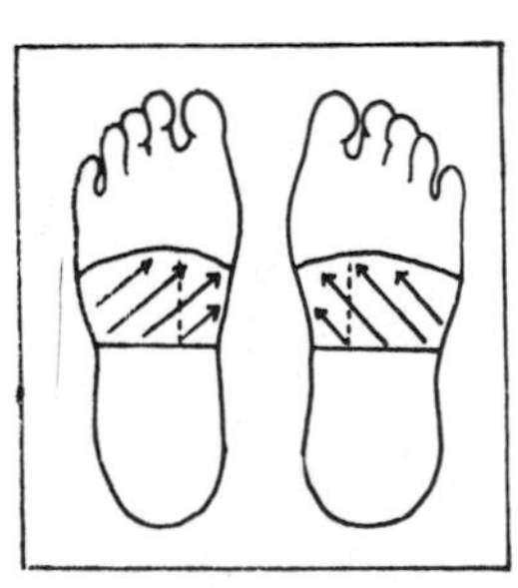

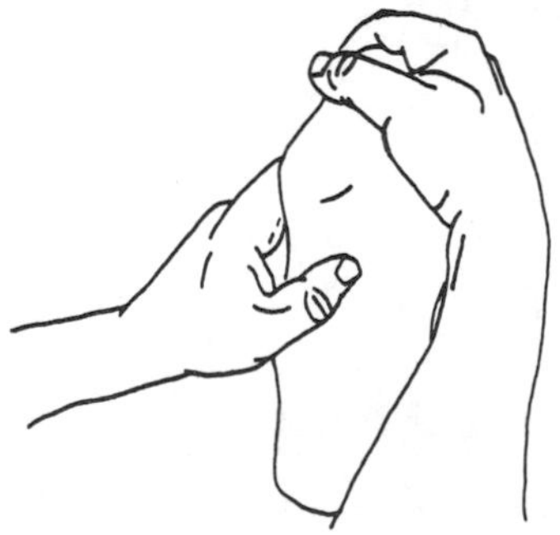

THE ARM AREA ON THE OUTSIDE OF THE FOOT: THUMB AND FINGER WALKING

arm
elbow
hand

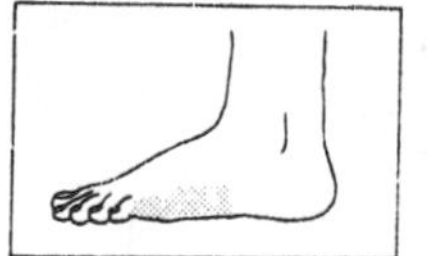

The arm reflex area runs from the base of the little toe to the 5th metatarsal bone along the outside edge of the foot. In reflex terms this means that it runs from the neck area to the waistline off of the shoulder, as the arm does on the body. The area between the neck and diaphragm generally corresponds to the upper arm; between the diaphragm and waistline (and even into the knee/leg area) corresponds to the elbow/forearm/hand.

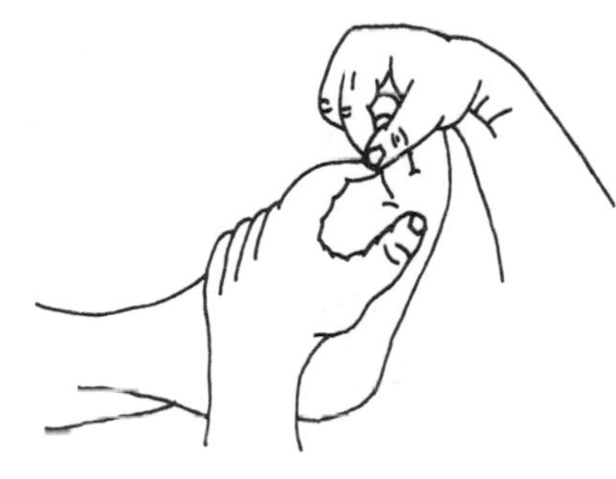

To work this area on the right foot, hold the foot with the right hand. Place the fingers of the left hand on top of the foot for leverage. Walk the thumb around the outside of the foot. Make several passes, covering this entire area. Change hands and, using the thumb of the right hand, walk around from the other direction. (See Illus.) Repeat for left foot, reversing hands.
Note: While it is possible to work the area by walking the thumb *up and down* the edge of the foot, it is somewhat more difficult because the foot is harder to hold comfortably.

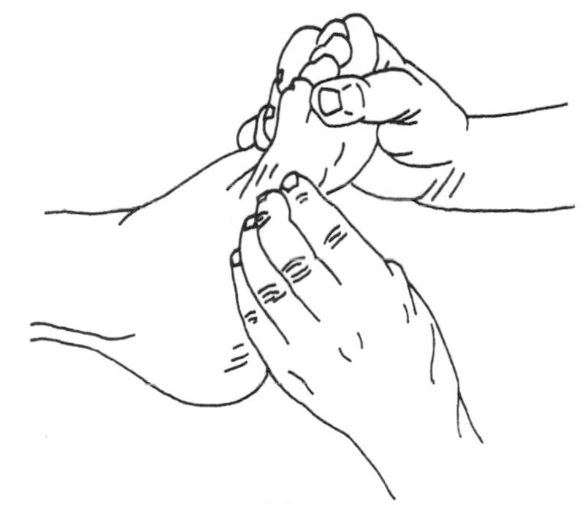

For fine tuning, walk the fingers (index and/or third) through the same area. Do so by first holding the right foot in the right hand, placing the thumb of the left hand on the bottom of the foot for leverage. Once again, make several passes in order to cover the whole area. In this instance, the fingers may have an advantage by enabling you to search out the nooks and crannies of the bones in this area, especially those of the 5th metatarsal. To walk the fingers through this area on the left foot, reverse hands and repeat the procedure.

BELOW THE WAISTLINE ON THE BOTTOM OF THE FOOT: THUMB WALKING

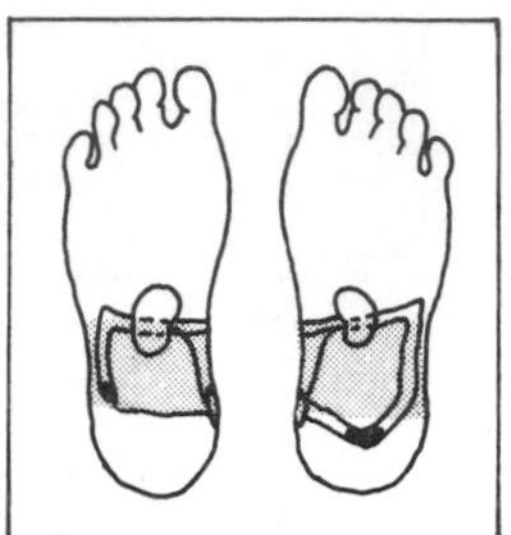

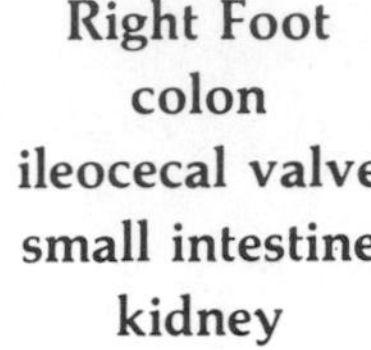

Right Foot	Left Foot
colon	colon
ileocecal valve	sigmoid colon
small intestine	small intestine
kidney	kidney

On the right foot this area includes the kidney, half of the small intestine framed by the colon, and the ileocecal valve. The ileocecal valve, which is located at the beginning of the colon, is worked by *pinpointing.* The rest of the area is criss-crossed using the *thumb walking* technique.

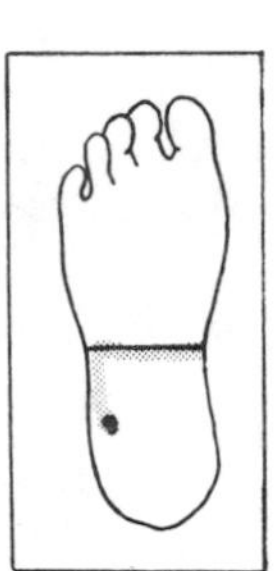

Begin by locating the ileocecal valve. It lies between the small and the large intestine areas. This area of the colon around the valve is responsible for the elimination of mucus. If it is not doing its job properly, the mucus is absorbed into the bloodstream and makes its way to other parts of the body. The sinuses are a likely spot. For a sinus problem, as well as any mucus problem, the ileocecal valve is an important area to work.

Look at the right foot. Try to visualize the intestines superimposed on it. The waistline bone, the 5th metatarsal, is a helpful reference point. Find the bone and the waistline. The transverse colon runs along this line. Starting at the 5th metatarsal, the ascending colon runs along the foot toward the heel.

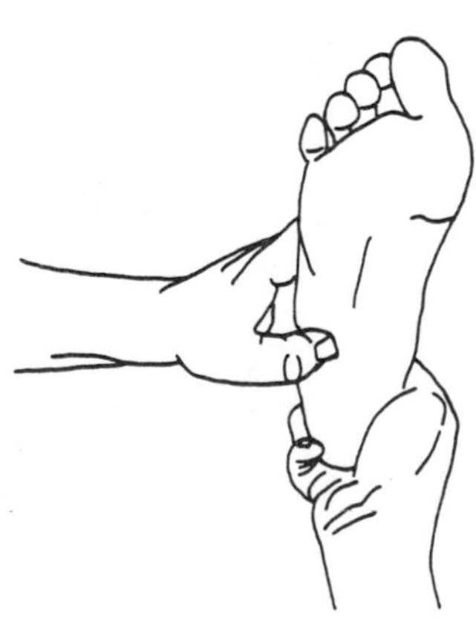

To find the ileocecal valve reflex point, run your hand down the outside of the foot from the 5th metatarsal bone to the heel. Do you feel the hollow spot along here? It is in the deepest part of this hollow that the valve is located. (See Illus.) Hook into this spot and back across it with your thumb. Once again, the fingers provide the all important leverage.

It may be difficult at first to break through the area,

so walk through it with the thumb from several directions.

This is a difficult technique to master. Some people become lazy and attempt to use the knuckle to penetrate the point. This is improper and dangerous. As we have stated, the knuckle has little feeling and therefore can not be controlled properly to prevent unnecessary pain or possible bruising.

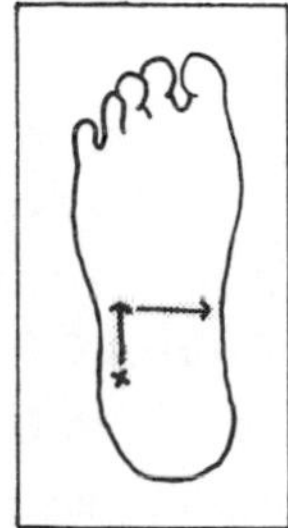

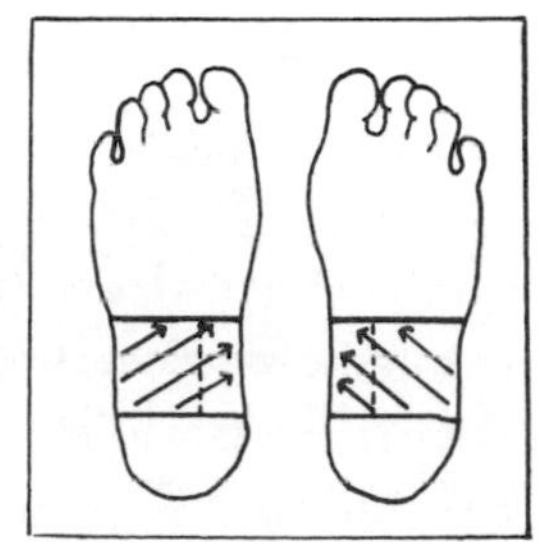

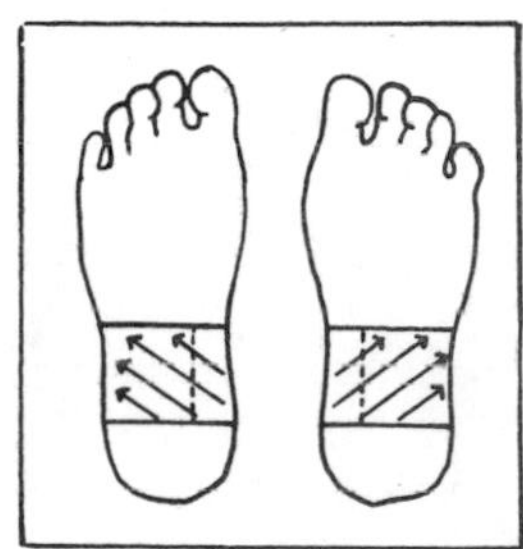

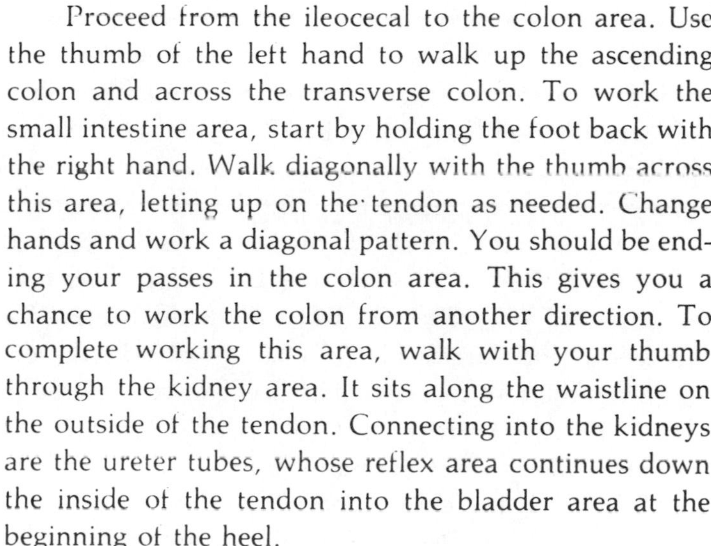

Proceed from the ileocecal to the colon area. Use the thumb of the left hand to walk up the ascending colon and across the transverse colon. To work the small intestine area, start by holding the foot back with the right hand. Walk diagonally with the thumb across this area, letting up on the tendon as needed. Change hands and work a diagonal pattern. You should be ending your passes in the colon area. This gives you a chance to work the colon from another direction. To complete working this area, walk with your thumb through the kidney area. It sits along the waistline on the outside of the tendon. Connecting into the kidneys are the ureter tubes, whose reflex area continues down the inside of the tendon into the bladder area at the beginning of the heel.

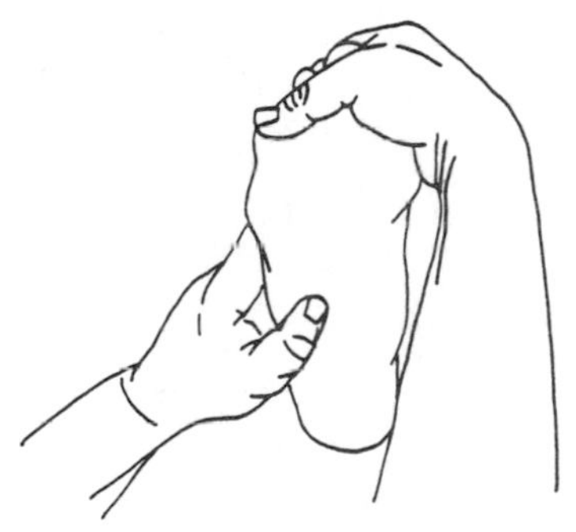

Since we have already walked through much of the kidney area when we criss-crossed the above-the-waist section, it is important not to assume the kidneys have been completely worked. They are important enough to be walked through from several directions. So hold the foot back with your right hand and walk up the outside of the tendon.

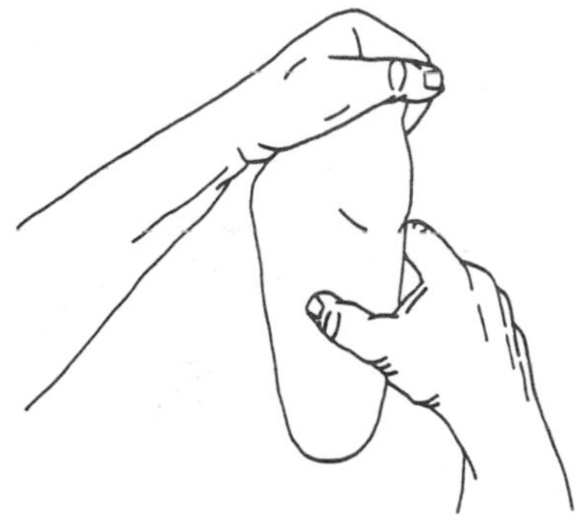

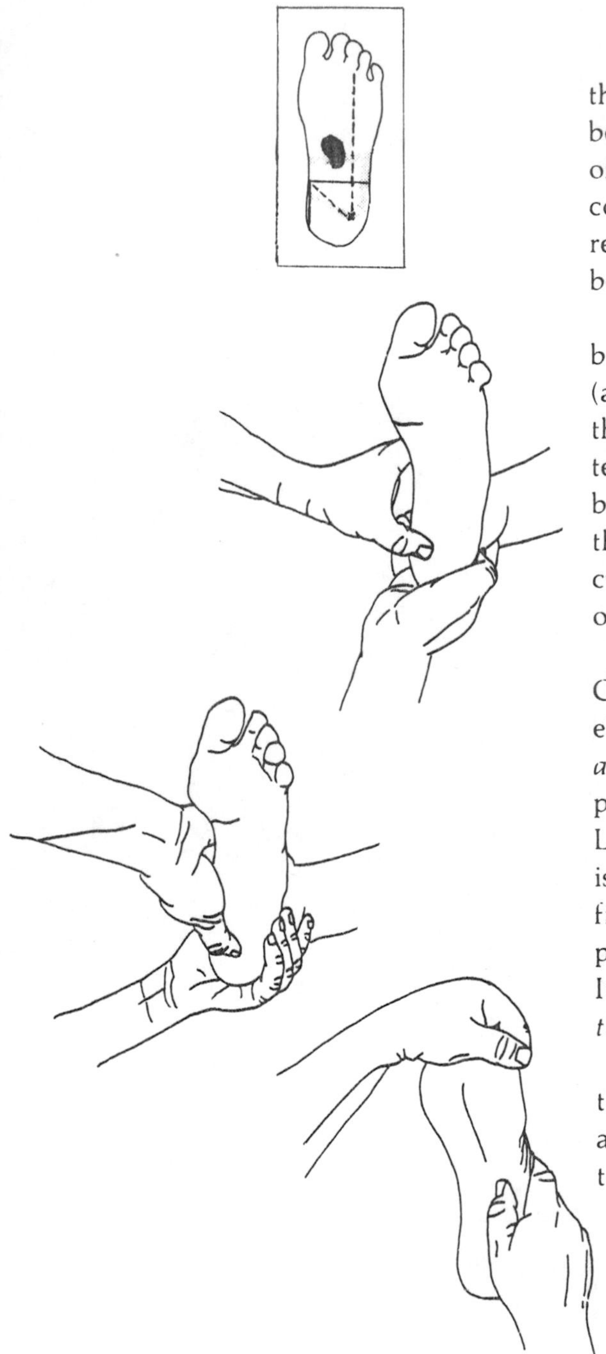

On the left foot, the kidney and the other half of the colon and small intestine are included in the area to be worked. Of special interest is a very important part of the colon, the sigmoid.This S-shaped section of the colon is the last turn before the wastes empty into the rectum for disposal. Because of its position, gas can become trapped here.

First, get an idea of its location. Draw a line on the bottom of the foot across the front edge of the heel (arch). Then draw another line along the inside edge of the heel, also on the bottom of the foot. This should intersect the first line (See Illus.) and form the corner of a box. From this corner, draw a line across the bottom of the heel itself at a 45° angle. The deepest part of the curve in the sigmoid colon is located three to three and one half zones in from this corner along the 45° line.

There are two ways to work this point. (See Illus.) Choose the one that works best for you. You can use either thumb to walk down the 45° line. Use the *hook and back up* technique to pinpoint the area. If anchored properly, a great deal of pressure can be applied. Leverage is the key to penetrating this point. If the hand is anchored properly you can pull with the leverage fingers as the thumb hooks. This is the most difficult point on the foot to reach. The heel can be very tough. It may require several passes from different directions of *thumb walking* just to loosen it up.

To work the colon areas of the left foot use the thumb of the right hand to walk up the descending colon and across the transverse colon. Work the small intestine and kidney just as you do on the right foot.

BELOW THE WAISTLINE ON THE TOP AND SIDES OF THE FEET: THUMB WALKING FINGER WALKING ROTATING ON A POINT

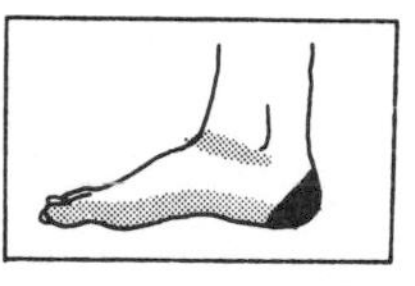

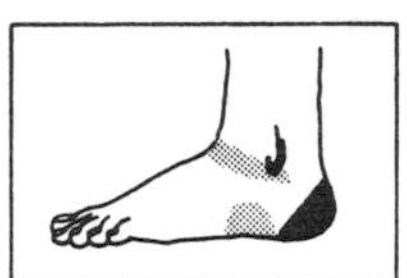

hip/sciatic
hip region
tailbone and spine
lymphatic/groin
hip joint (knee/leg)

This section of the foot contains reflex areas related to a host of health problems. Included among these are lower back, hip and tailbone disorders. Internal organs may be affected, such as problems with the colon or the reproductive organs. An injury to the tailbone can cause headaches (including migraines).

To understand how this area of the body corresponds to the feet, it is necessary to transpose the three-dimensional structure of the body to this particular portion of the foot. The spine is on the backside. The hip bone meets the spine and wraps around to the front of the body. What this means is that the top and sides of the feet contain important reflex areas directly related to this three-dimensional view of the lower back area of the body. This is a large area. You must use several different techniques to work it. The goal is to hit every single bit of the area.

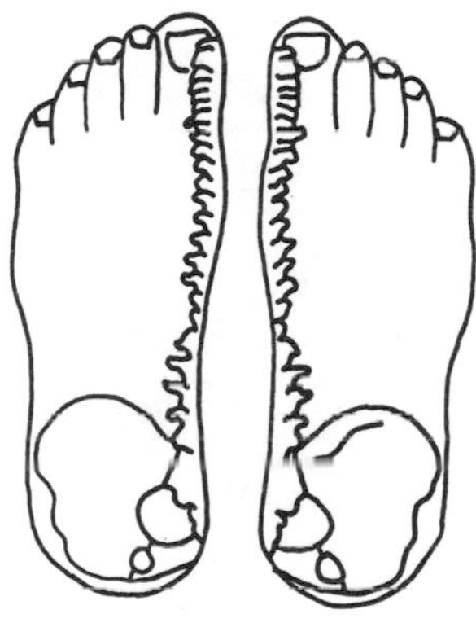

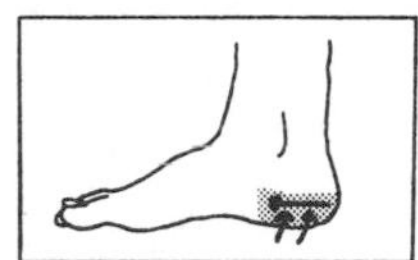

The tailbone and lower spine region is an area of the body prone to injury and stress. Often, injuries to the tailbone can be traced to childhood. Such an injury will make the corresponding area of the foot extremely sensitive. The area to be worked runs along the inside of the foot below the waistline well into the heel (See Illus.).

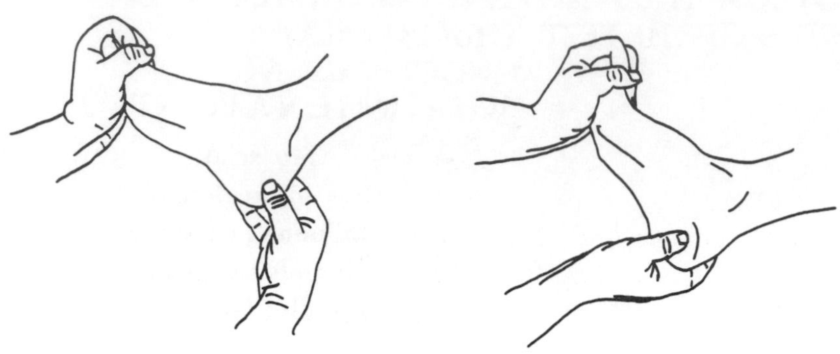

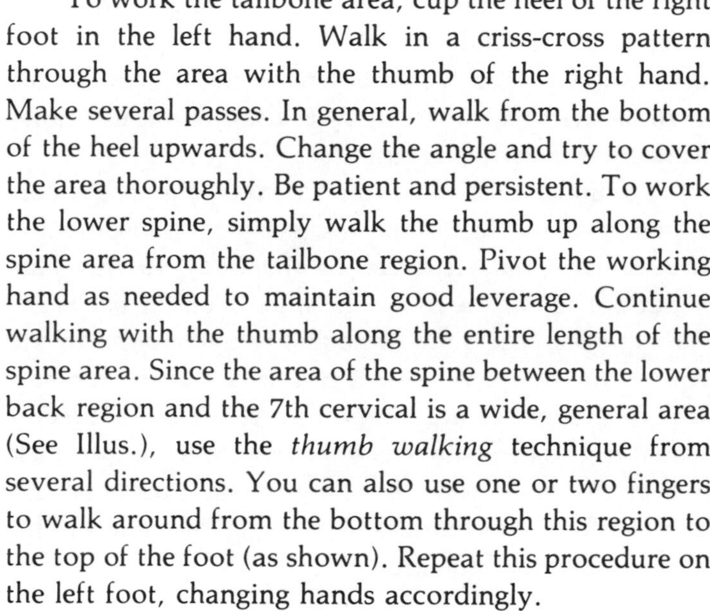

To work the tailbone area, cup the heel of the right foot in the left hand. Walk in a criss-cross pattern through the area with the thumb of the right hand. Make several passes. In general, walk from the bottom of the heel upwards. Change the angle and try to cover the area thoroughly. Be patient and persistent. To work the lower spine, simply walk the thumb up along the spine area from the tailbone region. Pivot the working hand as needed to maintain good leverage. Continue walking with the thumb along the entire length of the spine area. Since the area of the spine between the lower back region and the 7th cervical is a wide, general area (See Illus.), use the *thumb walking* technique from several directions. You can also use one or two fingers to walk around from the bottom through this region to the top of the foot (as shown). Repeat this procedure on the left foot, changing hands accordingly.

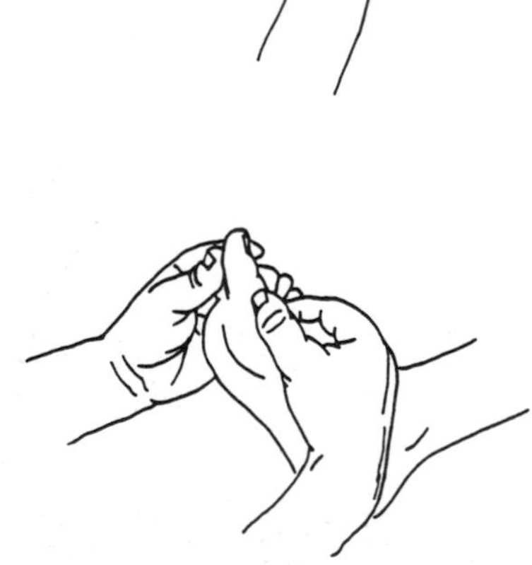

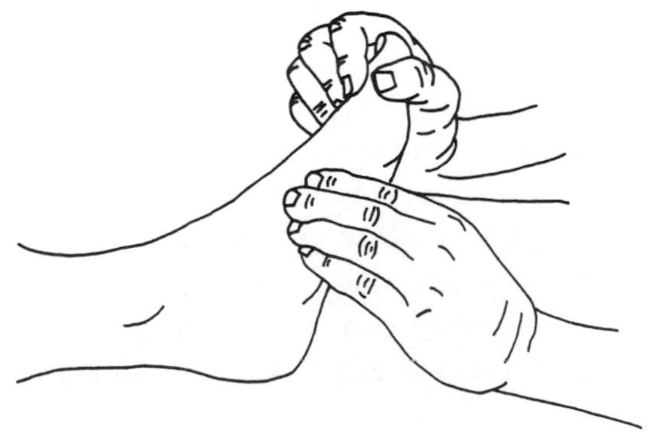

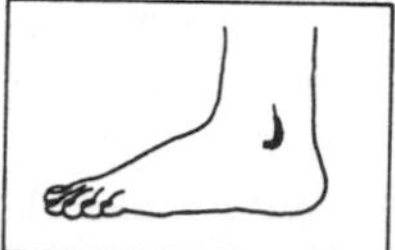

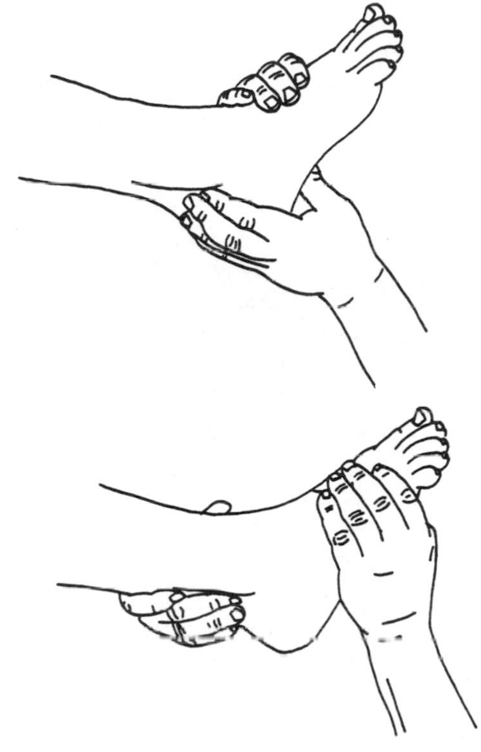

The region around the outside ankle bone should be the prime target when dealing with any hip or sciatic problem. Use the *finger walking* technique to walk around this area. The thumb is too awkward and difficult to control in this area.

Begin by cupping the right foot in your left hand. Use the index or third finger of the left hand to walk up through this area. Walk around the back of the ankle bone several times. When walking around the ankle bone, walk in the crease around it. If you walk short of this crease you'll hit the Achilles tendon, and if you overrun it you'll be hitting the ankle bone itself.

To complete the hip/sciatic area on the right foot, cup the right hand under the ankle and heel. Walk with the index or third finger of the left hand from the top of the foot down around the ankle bone (See Illus.). Be sure to hit the crease. Walking from the top of the foot down to the bottom of the ankle bone gives the deepest penetration.

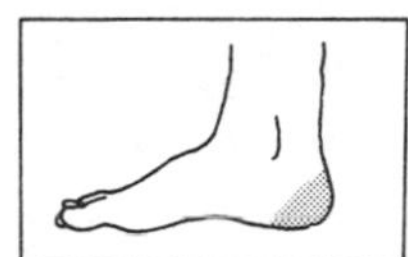

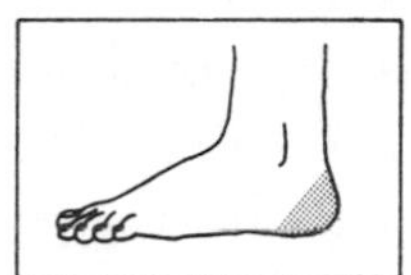

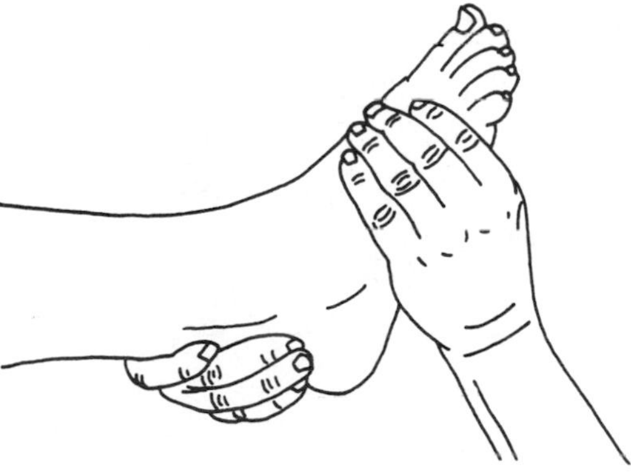

The hip region is often involved in lower back problems. (See Illus.) The reflex areas are found on the inside and outside of the foot. They are triangular in shape and are worked using the *finger walking* technique. To work these areas, cup the working hand around the back of the ankle. This provides leverage for the walking fingers. Walk down the area making several passes.

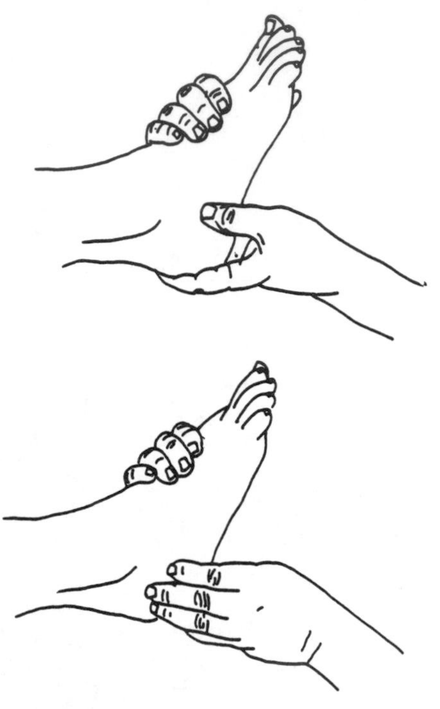

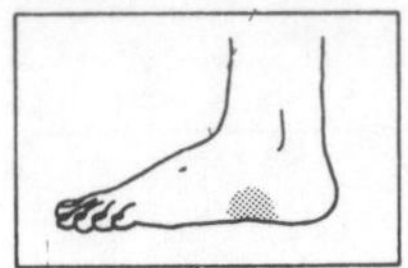

The area of the foot which actually corresponds to the hip joint has also been successfully worked for knee/thigh problems. These areas are linked by the muscles which originate around the hip bone and attach to the leg, including the knee. On the foot the area is bounded by the 5th metatarsal, the front edge of the heel on the bottom, and the boney area on the side of the foot.

Use either the *thumb* or *finger walking* technique to work the area. No particular precaution need be taken to hold the foot. Just keep the foot stationary. To use the thumb, plant the finger on the opposite side of the foot for leverage. Make several passes. Similarly, to walk with the finger through this area, plant the thumb on the bottom of the foot for leverage (as shown). Again, make several passes.

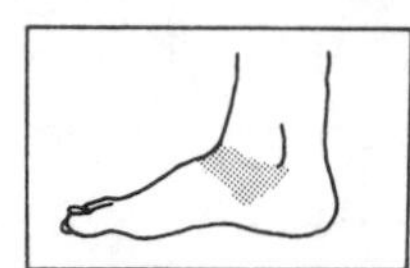

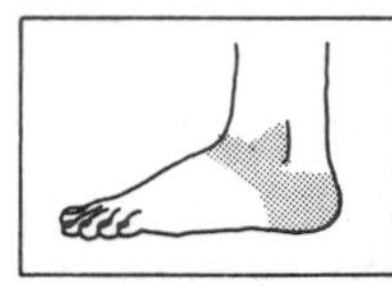

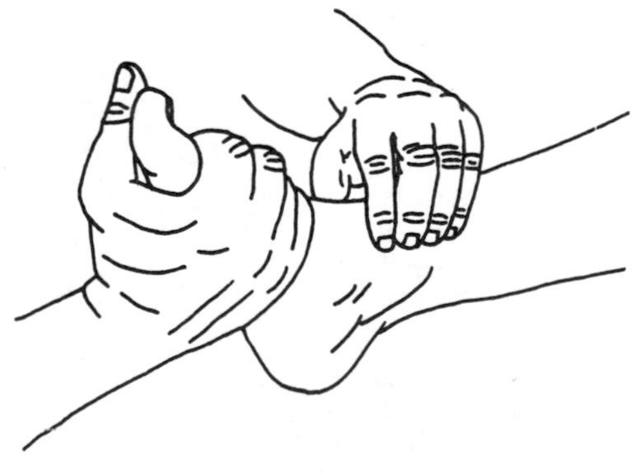

Rotating on a point is used to work the areas corresponding to the lower back region. Begin by *pinpointing* the areas described above (See Illus.). Notice that this is a boney region. The goal is to search the nooks and crannies of this region for sore points. When you find a sore point, exert pressure on it with the index finger. You can use other combinations of fingers but the index finger is able to exert the best pressure because of its ideal opposition to the thumb, the leverage giver.

Once you have located a sore point, apply the finger pressure. With the holding hand, grasp the foot below the base of the big toe on the inside of the foot. Rotate the foot with the holding hand. This will give a sense of increased pressure at the sore point. Shift the pressure finger around the region, exploring for other sore points. Rotate the foot in both directions at least five times. Don't dig with the fingernail. Of course, it is a good idea to keep your nails short enough to prevent any significant nail/skin contact. This technique is ideal for working on your own feet as well. If you wish, you can rotate your foot at the ankle without the aid of a holding hand. Just *pinpoint* the sore spots and turn the ankle in both directions.

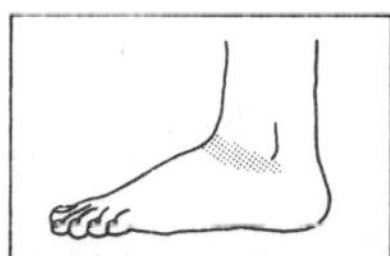
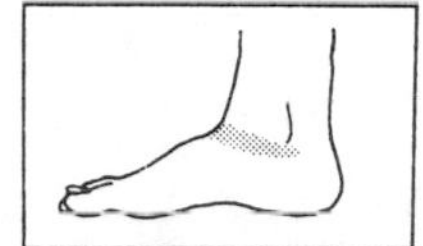

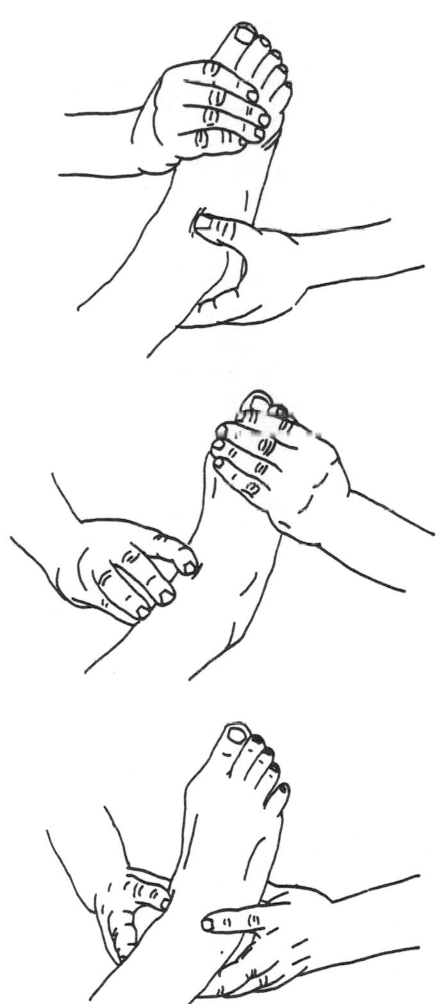

Most of the lymphatic nodes in the body are located in the groin, armpits and neck. Clustered in these locations, they protect the internal organs from infections in the extremeties. All five zones on both feet are affected by each of the three lymphatic areas. The region around the ankle encompasses all five zones and has been found to be effective in working on problems in any of the lymph glands. Included are the groin and the fallopian tubes.

The area to be worked runs from inside ankle bone around the top of the foot (crease) to the outside ankle bone. (See Illus.) This crease can be worked as a wide area by making several passes. Particular emphasis must be given to the primary area (as shown). To work with the thumb, hold the foot upright and stationary. Wrap the fingers of the working hand around the ankle and walk with the thumb along the crease. Change hands and walk with the other thumb from the opposite direction. To walk with the index finger (optional), use the same principles, using the thumb for leverage. You can also try walking both index fingers at the same time by placing the thumbs of both hands on the bottom of the foot and walking up on both sides until the two fingers meet in the middle, on the top of the foot.

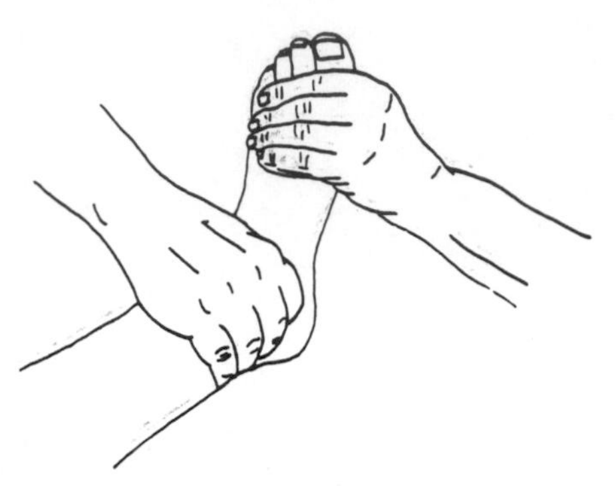

Swelling frequently affects this region because of lymph system problems. A little finesse can be applied when the area is sensitive to the touch. A *dessert* (See Illustration) can allow you to work the area in spite of the tenderness. Bridge your hand over the crease, fitting the thumb and first finger into the crease itself. Rotate the foot in both directions at least five times. (Generally the left hand works better bridging the right foot, etc.) You can also use the *rotating on a point* technique in the lymph area to locate and work sore points within it.

To work the left foot, repeat the above procedure exactly. Reverse hands when appropriate.

Reproductive System on the Sides of the Heel: Pinpointing

uterus/prostate
ovary/testicle

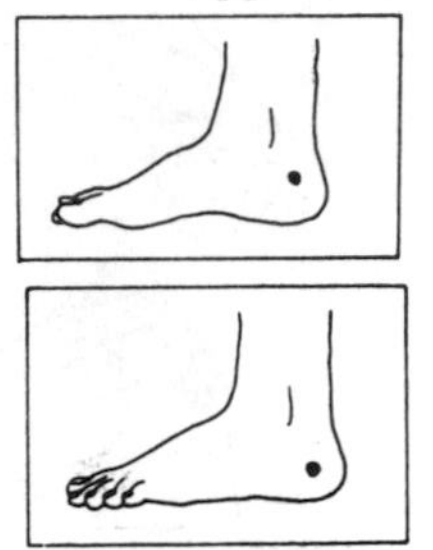

The uterus/prostate area is located on the inside of the foot below the ankle bone. It is a pinpoint area, so correctly locating it is crucial to effectively hitting the point. This area of the foot is commonly tender but this does not necessarily mean problems specific to the reproductive organs and glands. Working this area can be helpful, for example, in alleviating allergic reactions.

To *pinpoint* the area, place the tip of the index finger on the ankle bone (inside the foot) and the tip of the fourth finger on the back corner of the heel. Draw the third finger in until it forms a straight line with the others and establishes the midpoint. This is the uterus/prostate reflex area to be worked. (See Illus.)

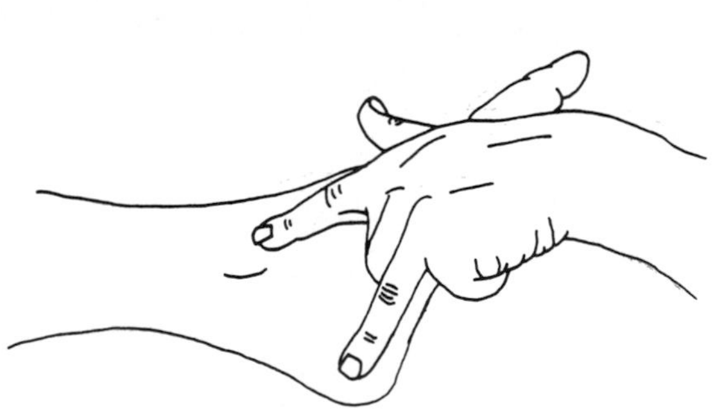

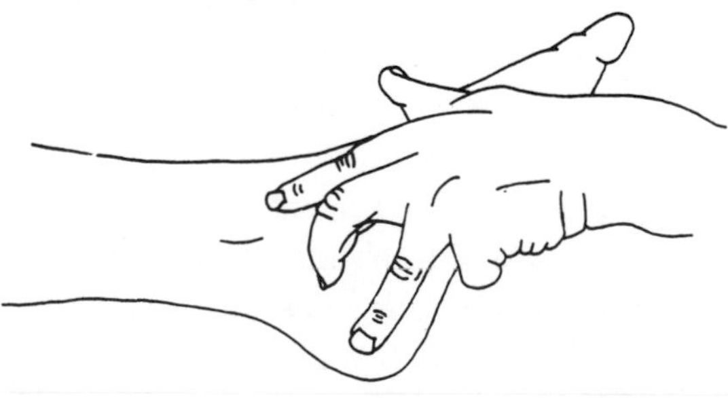

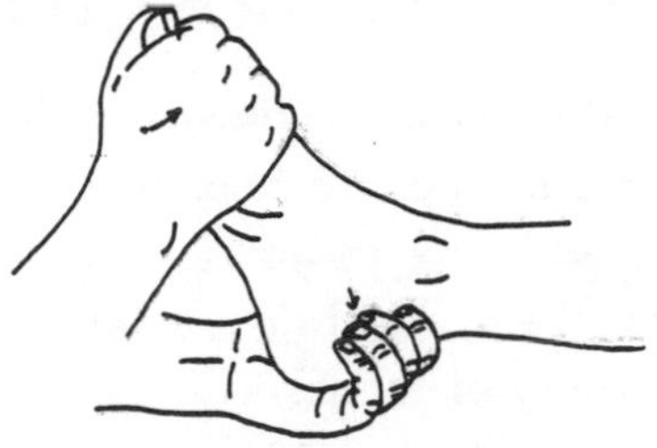

To work the area on the right foot, use the left hand. Cup the heel, curling the third finger in such a way as to place its tip on the point to be worked. The thumb should be positioned in the lymphatic area on the top of the foot. Now rotate the foot with the right hand in both directions several times. You can vary the amount of pressure you use with the third finger as appropriate. By *rotating on a point* you *pinpoint* accurately while limiting the amount of discomfort for your subject.

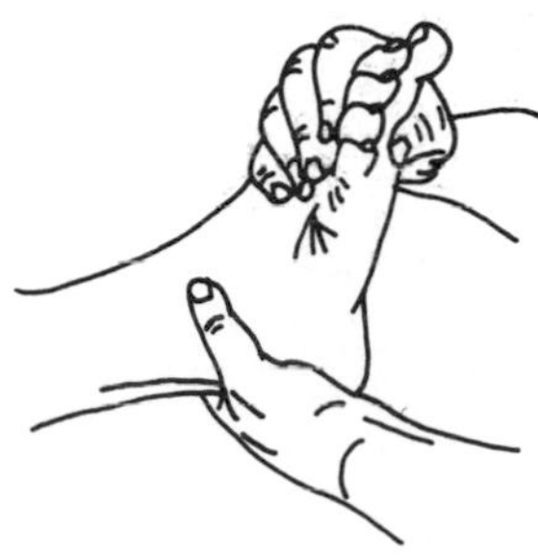

To work the left foot area, simply reverse hands and repeat the procedure.

To locate the ovary/testicle area use the same technique as you use for the uterus/prostate. (See Illus.) Since the area is on the boney outside of the foot walk through it with the thumb of the left hand. You can also walk the finger of the right hand through this area, holding the foot just as you do for working the hip/sciatic area.

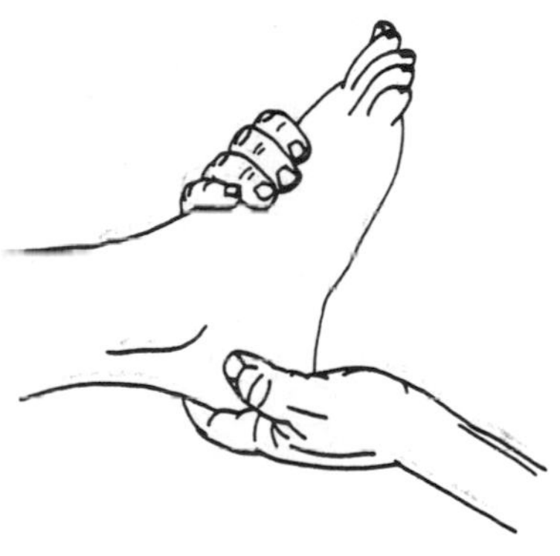

On the left foot, repeat the procedure, reversing hands.

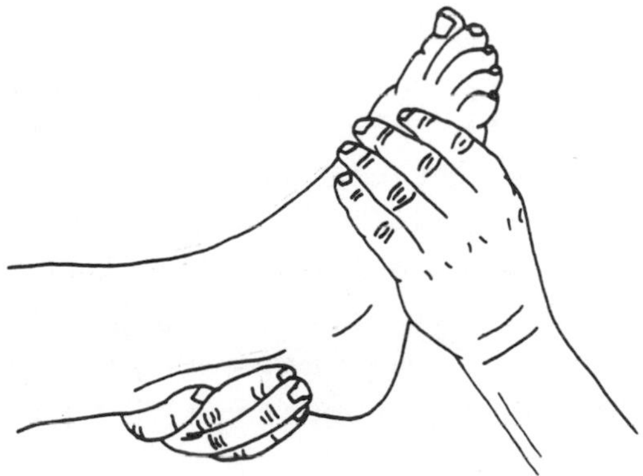

DESSERTS/RELAXATION TECHNIQUES

One of the primary goals of reflexology is to ease tension, to negate the effects of stress upon the body. In conjunction with the series of techniques discussed in this chapter, there are things a reflexologist can do to reduce sensitivity or tenderness in the feet. Not only will this relax your subject, it will open up the areas of the feet that need working. These supplemental techniques are called "desserts" for their relaxing and pleasure-giving qualities.

An effective treatment is one in which all important areas have been worked thoroughly while leaving the subject relaxed, with a feeling of well-being. Such treatment is administered by skillfully mixing in the desserts throughout, thereby maintaining the relaxing effect of the whole technique. While pain *is* a good indicator of problems, a road map that tells a reflexologist where to concentrate his efforts, it is by no means the objective. A skillful operator does not seek to GIVE pain, only to locate it, and, while keeping the subject comfortable and relaxed, to work the area while the desserts do their job.

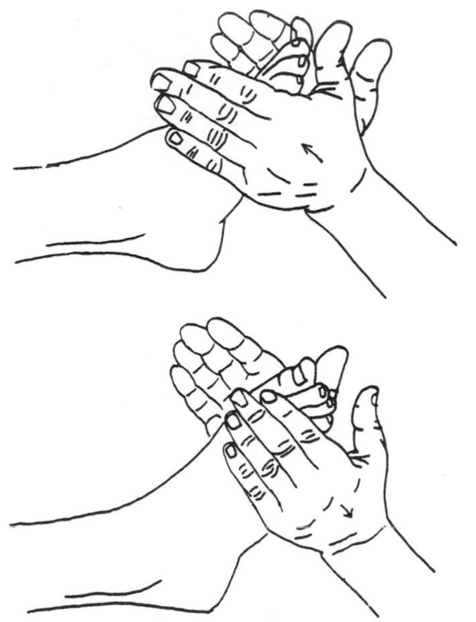

DESSERT NUMBER ONE: SIDE TO SIDE

This dessert is a way of vigorously shaking the foot to help circulation, ease tenderness, and relax the muscles of the ankle and calf. Place the hands on either side of the foot (as shown) The area of the hands right below the fingers should be in contact with the sides of the foot just below the toes.

With a vigorous motion rapidly work the foot back and forth, maintaining the hands in their starting position. When the right hand moves away the left hand draws toward you and so forth. It is a rapid rocking motion, however try to keep the hands as relaxed and loose as possible. Avoid attempting to force the foot to rotate farther than is comfortable for your subject. But do not relax too much or your hands will slip on the foot and render the dessert ineffective.

DESSERT NUMBER TWO: HOOK IN THE ANKLES

This dessert did not derive its name from a fishing accident,as rumor once had it. It is indeed a very relaxing technique if done properly. Hook the base of both palms above the back sides of the heel so that the palms themselves cover the ankle bones. Using an alternating movement similar to the *side to side* dessert, work the whole foot back and forth, with the ankle joint serving as the pivot point.

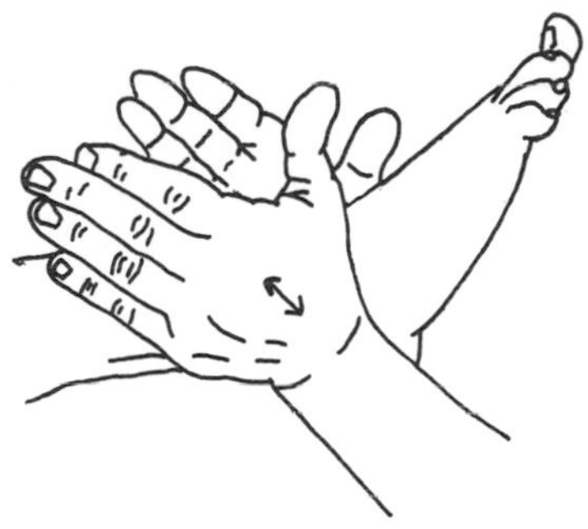

The key to this dessert is rapid, relaxed motion, keeping the palms secured in place around the ankle bones. You'll know you've got it when the foot wiggles back and forth in an almost blurred motion.

DESSERT NUMBER THREE: SPINAL TWIST

This is a delightful tension reducer. Place your hands around the foot so that the index fingers and thumbs are right next to each other. Position the hands so that the thumbs are on the bottom of the foot and the fingers grip the foot on top. Your hands should now be positioned so that, while index finger and thumbs are touching, the foot is being gripped on the inside, or arch side.

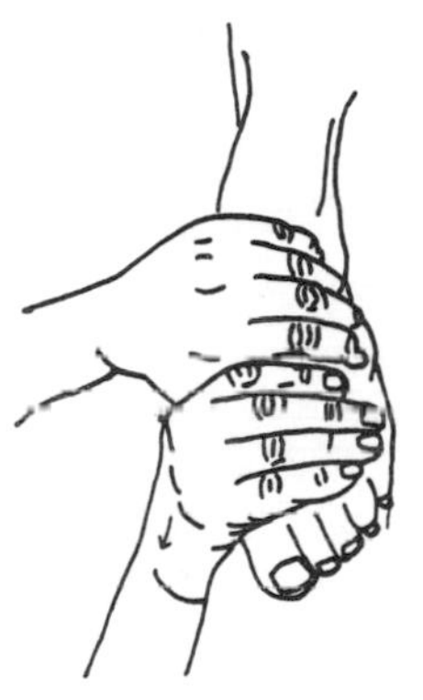

Now turn the hand nearest the toes while keeping the other stationary. Make a back-and-forth motion with the turning hand (imagine a wringing motion with one hand doing all the turning). Maintain an evenly distributed gripping pressure, just enough to hold the foot without letting the hands slip.

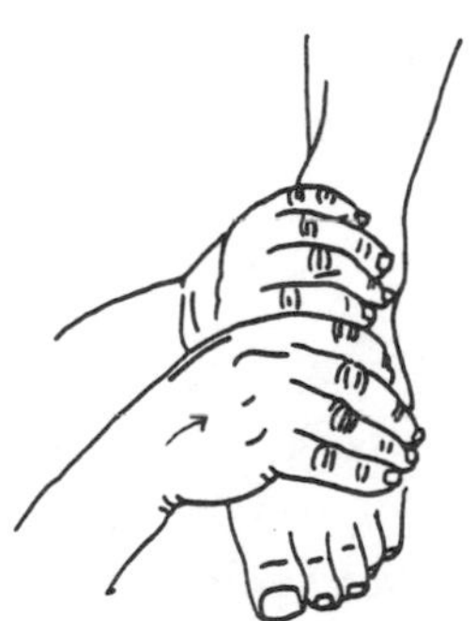

To apply this dessert to the foot, begin at the lower spine area. Make several turns of the hand nearest the toes keeping the other hand stationary. Then reposition both hands slightly closer to the toes and repeat. Continue in this manner (i.e. grip and twist, reposition, grip and twist, reposition, etc.) until the index finger of the twisting hand reaches the base area of the toes. Do not go into the toe area. Do not twist both hands at the same time. The attempt is to twist the foot around the spine area (see foot chart), *not* to impart a wringing sensation to the whole foot. You can repeat the spinal twist dessert as desired.

DESSERT NUMBER FOUR: ANKLE ROTATION

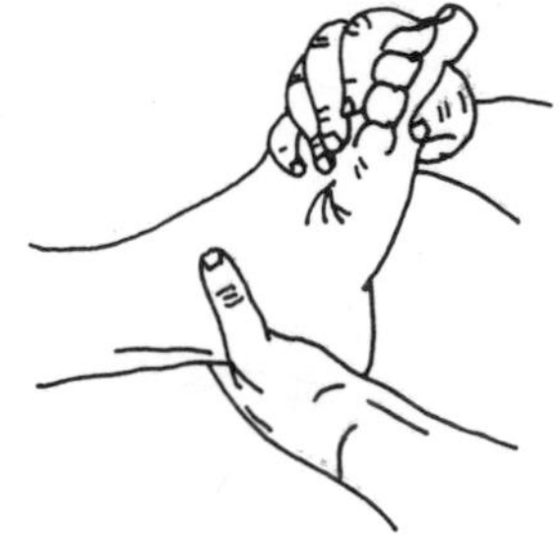

This dessert is designed to provide a precise method for rotating the ankles. It is not as simple as just grabbing the foot and turning it. This would surely be ineffective and the ankle joint would not be properly rotated.

Use the left hand to grasp the right foot around the ankle and vice versa. Wrap the fingers around the heel so that the thumb rests in the lymphatic area on top. Grasp with even pressure. With the other hand grasp the foot below the base of the big toe on the inside of the foot. Once again use even pressure when holding the foot. Now rotate the foot in full 360° circles, using the hand holding the heel as a pivot point. Try to sense what the ankle joint is doing as you rotate with your top hand. Maintain constant pressure throughout each rotation. Rotate in both directions. Do not grasp the toes. Make smooth, firm rotations.

DESSERT NUMBER FIVE: LUNG PRESS

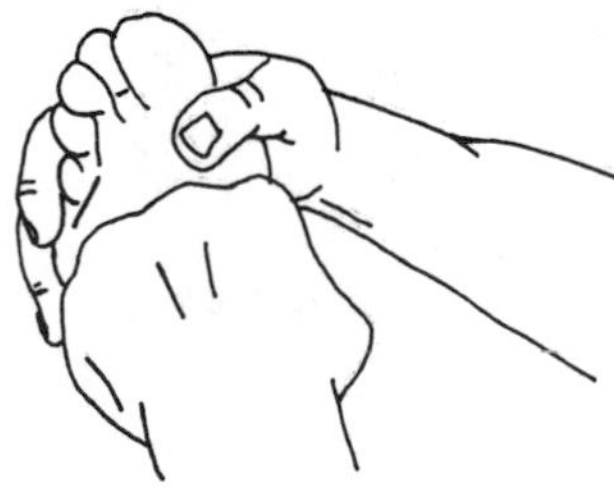

There is an art to this dessert. It may look easy but it really takes a bit of coordination and a good deal of finesse. Properly done it can be extremely comforting especially for people with lung-related problems.

Make a fist. For the right foot use the left hand for the fist. Place the fist on the bottom of the foot in the lung area as if you were punching the foot.(See Illus.)

With the right hand across the lung area on top of the foot, curve it slightly around the foot so that the fingers are on top and can reach slightly around the outside edge of the foot.

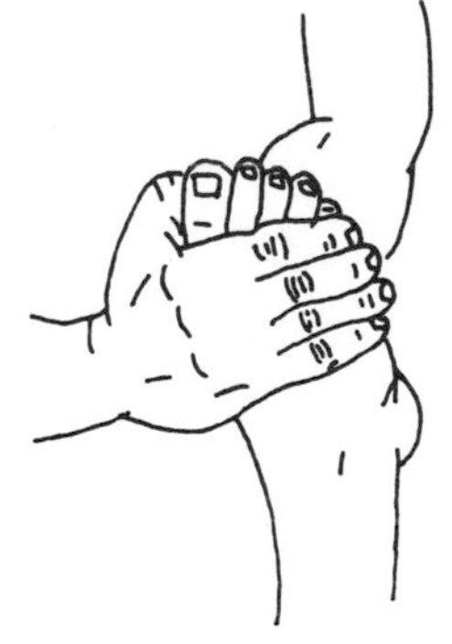

Press in with the fist against the foot, using the right hand as a backstop. As you let up on this pressure, squeeze with the right hand and push with it back toward the fist. Now the fist is the backstop. The combination of these two pushing motions with the squeezing of the right hand gives a kind of kneading effect. A smooth, wavelike motion is the goal. Think of a wave breaking on the shore. The hands answer each other with pushing motions. The hand on top of the foot has the trickiest part, having to push and squeeze at the same time.

This is not a forceful dessert. It is designed to work the ball of the foot in a pleasure-giving way. With practice the technique becomes most soothing for your subject.

To work the left foot, reverse hands. You can use the opposite hands on either foot if there is a sensitive bunion in the way.

DESSERT NUMBER SIX: TOE ROTATION

The principles of *toe rotation* are identical to those of *ankle rotation.* The goal is the same for the joints of the toes as it is for the ankles during *ankle rotation*.

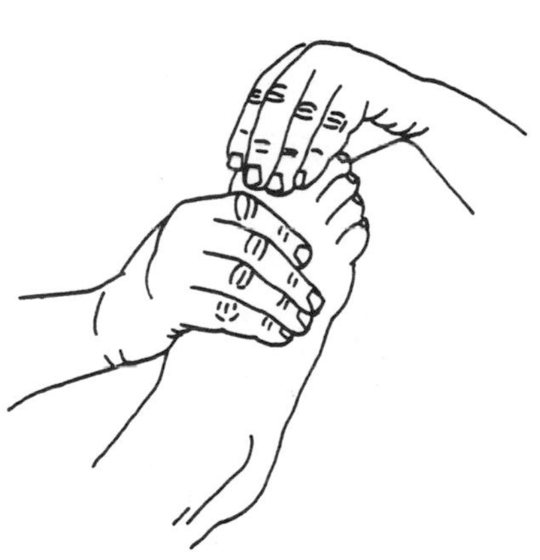

Place the fingers on the toe (as shown). The fingertips should extend almost to the base of the toe. Using firm, even pressure with the grasping fingers and a slight upward pull, rotate the toe slowly and evenly in full 360° turns. Rotate in both directions several times.

The big toe, of course, is the main center of attraction here but the little toes can be rotated as well. In general, use the fingers of the right hand for rotating the toes of the right foot and so forth. Done properly, this dessert is soothing and effective.

DESSERT NUMBER SEVEN: THE FEATHERING TOUCH

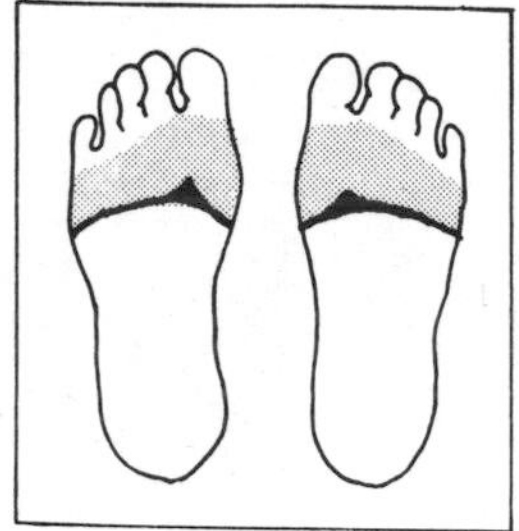

If stress is the Goliath among sources of physical problems, this dessert is the David that will bring it down. It is particularly effective when applied to the solar plexus/diaphragm area on the bottom of the foot. But it can also be used on the toes (neck, head/sinus) and lymphatic/groin area.

Essentially the *feathering touch* describes itself very well. It is a light, rhythmic motion using the *thumb walking* technique. The basic idea is to walk very lightly and rapidly through the area to be *feathered.*

To *feather* the solar plexus/diaphragm area, do not try to hit the reflex points per se. Cover the entire area by starting down in the solar plexus region and *feathering* up through the lung area. Do not concern yourself with the troughs. Work lightly and smoothly, repeatedly walking through the entire region from bottom to top. Since this area is the main storage center for stress in the body, the effect of this dessert should be immediately apparent on the face of your subject. Watch his/her expressions to find the areas or *feathering* techniques which are most pleasing.

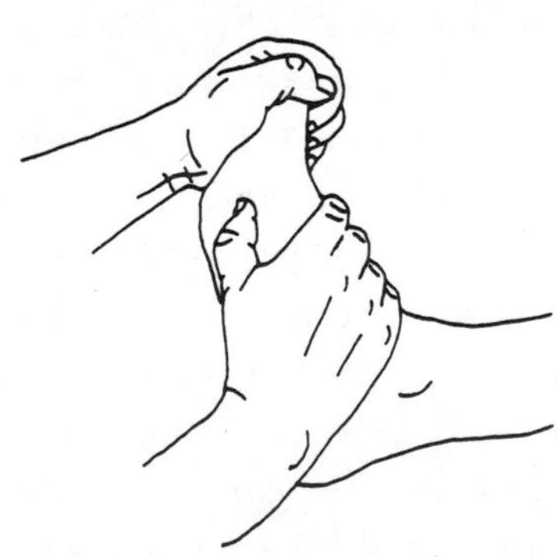

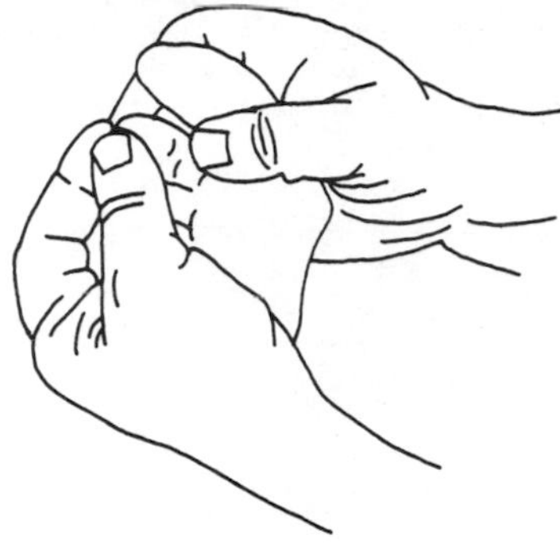

To *feather* the toes, walk up them with the thumb lightly. Use quick, gentle motions. If the toes are short or thick, they may be difficult to *feather* with the thumb — do not struggle with them. Simply walk up the sides, or find other areas to *feather*. Remember: the idea is to give pleasure and to relax your subject.

You can *feather* your thumb through the lymphatic/groin area as well as the general lower back region of the foot. The lymphatic area lends itself nicely to rapid strokes delivered by the fingers too. Put the finishing touches on with rapid, delicate *feathering* with the fingers (as shown).

This dessert requires some restraint. Reflexologists tend to equate progress with breaking down deposits. This, of course, implies the use of varying amounts of pressure. But many times, part of the pain or sensitivity which puts resistance between your pressure and those deposits is due directly to tension or stress. Five minutes of *feathering* can relax your subject so profoundly that it may actually make his/her feet less sensitive to the pressure of normal techniques. And the bottom line is, of course: a relaxed subject will enjoy *and* benefit from the treatment.

The Treatment

SUGGESTED TREATMENT PATTERN

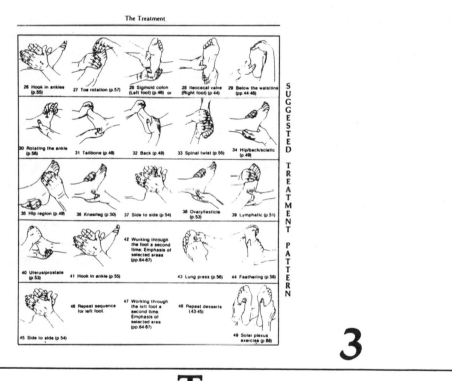

26 Hook in ankles (p.55)	27 Toe rotation (p.57)	28 Sigmoid colon (Left foot) (p.46) or	28 Ileocecal valve (Right foot) (p.44)	29 Below the waistline (pp.44-46)
30 Rotating the ankle (p.56)	31 Tailbone (p.48)	32 Back (p.48)	33 Spinal twist (p.55)	34 Hip/back/sciatic (p.49)
35 Hip region (p.49)	36 Knee/leg (p.50)	37 Side to side (p.54)	38 Ovary/testicle (p.53)	39 Lymphatic (p.51)
40 Uterus/prostate (p.53)	41 Hook in ankle (p.55)	42 Working through the foot a second time: Emphasis of selected areas (pp.64-67)	43 Lung press (p.56)	44 Feathering (p.58)
45 Side to side (p.54)	46 Repeat sequence for left foot.	47 Working through the left foot a second time. Emphasis of selected area (pp.64-67)	48 Repeat desserts (43-45)	49 Solar plexus exercise (p.68)

3

The Treatment

THE TREATMENT

Putting the techniques together into a coherent pattern is in itself a part of reflexology. The techniques (Chapter 2) provide the most effective and efficient way of working each area. The goal of the treatment is to combine the techniques into an organized and consistent pattern to get the best results and at the same time make it a relaxing experience for your client.

The pattern is a systematic, repeatable method of working the areas on the feet. We suggest working through the foot twice. The first time through covers every area on the foot, while the second emphasizes key areas as needed by each individual. Working every single area at least once is necessary because reflexology deals with the body as a whole. Working only the shoulder area for a shoulder problem ignores its possible connection to the neck and back, whose areas can be related to the problem and can be worked in conjunction with it. In other words, working all areas serves to amplify your efforts on any one problem.

It is your choice as to which areas to emphasize during the second time through each foot. This is what makes reflexology so interesting. But it takes practice and training. You will be involved in a constant re-evaluation of each foot to see where you are achieving the desired results.

GETTING STARTED

Start the treatment with either foot. Beginning with right or left is a matter of personal preference. But be consistent with each individual. It is important, however, to work thoroughly the foot you start with. Switching from one foot to the other is not as relaxing for your subject. It also makes it more difficult to remember which areas you have worked and which need emphasis on the second time through.

Working through every single area at least once does not mean that your thumb makes contact with each area of the foot *only* once. When you work an area, make several passes through it. The sample pattern (See Illus., pg. 70) shows the pituitary area to be worked. You should hit the pituitary not once but several times.

To achieve continuity in your techniques, use the desserts. (See pg. 54). Also, at all times keep at least one hand on the foot on which you are working. In most cases this will be the holding hand because you will constantly be repositioning the working hand to work other areas.

Our pattern suggestion starts with the toes and works through the foot to the heel. It is not necessary to follow this exact sequence. Develop one with which you will be comfortable. But remember to include the desserts and work through every area in each foot at least once.

At first, if you try to stick with one technique too long, your thumb or fingers may get tired. Learn how to vary your techniques to avoid fatigue. For example, when the walking thumb begins to tire, change to a dessert, or switch hands and walk with the other thumb from the opposite direction. As you build your hand strength over a period of time, this will be less of a concern.

EVALUATING THE FOOT

Just as an artist highlights certain areas in a painting, the reflexologist identifies and highlights areas on the feet. The second time through the foot is your opportunity to emphasize key and selected areas. This is the "evaluation" phase of the treatment and is the real heart of your effectiveness and efficiency. Your ability to evaluate will determine the degree to which you get results.

Key areas are those corresponding to organs, such as the endocrine glands and the spine (as representative of the central nervous system), that regulate the major functions of the body. These areas may overlap with the selected areas but their importance is such that they require emphasis regardless of your evaluation. The areas you "select" are chosen as a result of your evaluation.

It will require time and practice to master the evaluation process. Thinking through a problem is a necessity. It pays to know where to look and to have several ready references to understand the problem. After all, in emphasizing areas the goal is to maximize results with your most efficient effort. If the areas you have selected during your evaluation do not prove successful over time, a re-analysis of your pattern is necessary. A shift in emphasis may improve results. Explore each foot, keep an open mind, and constantly re-evaluate.

There are criteria to guide your selection of areas for emphasis. If your client declares a specific problem, refer to the Tables (pages 108 to 142). If the problem is listed alphabetically in the "Table", note the cross references and directions on techniques. If it's not listed, refer to the Anatomy Section for general information on the part of the body affected. Search through the suggested areas totally. Do not neglect the tops and sides of the feet. The Table only gives you a place to start. The feedback that you get from the actual feet will guide you more accurately. After all, symptomatic complaints are frequently misleading. The root cause may seem to be unconnected to the symptom.

Here are some guidelines to enhance your effectiveness on problems that may not be listed in the Table of Disorders. Always suspect stress as a root cause (See pg. 15). It has been implicated in the majority of disorders. Work through the solar plexus/diaphragm area again and again using the feathering technique (See pg. 58). If there is a buildup or problem in an area, check the entire zone on the foot looking for sensitivity or buildup. These areas can be the root cause of the initial problem or they can at least contribute to it.

TOUCH AS AN EVALUATIVE TOOL

Evaluation involves observation of areas of buildup on the feet. The buildup consists of deposits of calcium or lymph fluid (see pg. 17). Buildup in any area needs to be worked. Not all of the areas needing work will be indicated by buildup so the guidelines for evaluation should always be followed.

Developing the ability to detect changes in the texture and condition of a foot is a vital component of every reflexologist's training. Some calcium deposits such as those at the base of the toes are hard and thus difficult to distinguish from the bone. Other deposits are soft and puffy.

Like other techniques and skills in reflexology, feeling for buildup requires practice and, in this case, observation. Compare your feet with a friend's. Evaluate the toes. Do your toes feel exactly the same to the touch as your friends? Look for any puffiness. Do both pair of feet have exactly the same puffiness in the same places?

Detecting this buildup is essential to your evaluation. The purpose is not to alarm the person you are working on. Buildup in an area indicates congestion which needs to be broken down. It should be considered in the context of the whole zone.

EVALUATION THROUGH SYSTEMS

There are many health problems that involve general body systems. They fall into general categories because they are seldom isolated to one specific area. The systems involved are the hormonal (endocrine), the digestive, the nervous, the cardio-vascular, the lymphatic, the respiratory, the urinary, the reproductive, the skeletal and the muscular.

Often your client will have a medical diagnosis of his or her problem and you can use a medical dictionary to find out which system is affected. At other times it may be necessary to identify the system based on the *nature* of the problems as described by the client.

For example, check all reflex areas of the digestive system for a problem in any of the areas listed for that system. The table below is very helpful:

SYSTEMS	ORGANS or GLANDS
ENDOCRINE	Pituitary, Adrenal Glands, Pancreas, Ovary/Testicle, Uterus/Prostate
DIGESTIVE	Stomach, Gallbladder, Liver, Pancreas, Small Intestine, Large Intestine
URINARY	Kidneys, Ureter Tubes, Bladder
REPRODUCTIVE	Ovary, Uterus, Fallopian Tubes (for females) Testicles, Prostate (for males)
NERVOUS	Spinal Cord, Brain
CIRCULATORY	Heart, Arteries, Veins
LYMPHATIC	Lymph Ducts, Spleen, Thymus
RESPIRATORY	Lung

The skeletal and muscular systems cover the entire body. Stress contributes to their problems and disorders. If a specific muscle or bone is affected, use referral areas (see pg. 12) and/or find the corresponding area on the foot. This can require some searching.

As the body's framework, the skeletal system requires special consideration. The neck is a crossroad for shoulders, arms and head. Check it for problems in these areas. The lower back affects everything in that area including digestion, reproduction and lower limbs. It can be a helper for or root cause of many problems in that region of the body.

EVALUATION OF ACTUAL FOOT PROBLEMS

Take note of foot problems such as corns, calluses, ingrown or thickened toe nails, bunions and displaced bones. They put direct pressure on an area of the foot which will affect the corresponding part of the body.

The foot problem must be dealt with to eliminate the negative effects on the body (See pg. 17).

THE RELAXATION ASPECT

You work with a person, not just a pair of feet. Your client's comfort during the treatment is a very important element. The pressure you exert should be attuned to the subject's tolerance level. As a matter of fact, the pressure you use will change many times during the course of a treatment. Some areas on a person's feet will be more sensitive than others. Relaxation is not achieved with just a few desserts. Working to the client's tolerance point rather than past the threshold of pain contributes to the overall feeling of relaxation and trust he or she should have at the end of the treatment.

There are several ways to judge a person's tolerance level. Keep your eyes on the face. The most obvious sign of discomfort will be registered in facial expressions. Also the feet themselves may stiffen or jerk with pain. If you are in doubt ask the person whether you are using too much pressure. Do not assume that one foot will have the same degree of sensitivity as the other. The sensitivity of feet also varies from treatment to treatment. You should always be alert to the effects your work is having.

Remember: your goal as a reflexologist is to cover all the areas effectively, yet give the person a feeling of relaxation.

RELAXATION EXERCISE (Solar Plexus)

This exercise is one designed primarily for relaxation and can be an excellent way of signaling the end of the treatment. Place the fingers of each hand on the tops of the feet for leverage. Place both thumbs in the hollow between the big toe and the second toe below the ball of the foot. This is the solar plexus/diaphragm area.

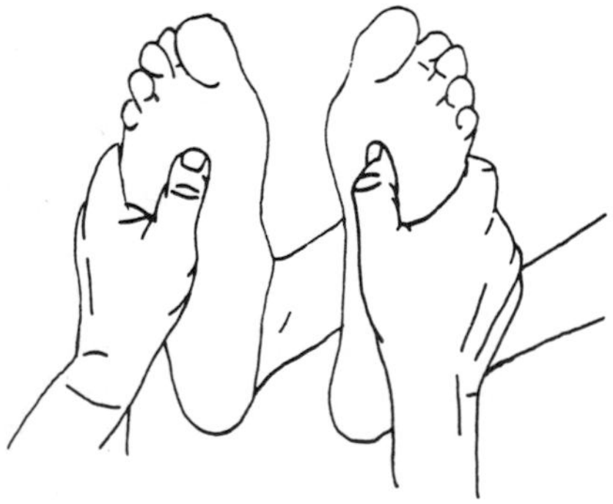

Explain to the person that this is a relaxation exercise. Ask your client to take four deep breaths (more if you think it necessary) while you exert a straight inward pressure on both thumbs. Keep the pressure constant but comfortable throughout the breathing. On the last exhalation, gradually release the thumb pressure. It can also be relaxing and reassuring if you will breathe along with your client during this final exercise.

SELF-HELP

Homework is an assigned program of self-help techniques so that your client can work selected areas between treatments. The value of homework is twofold: it encourages individuals to get involved in their own health and it speeds up results. Your client may or may not be interested in learning everything about reflexology or the techniques. The techniques are the most efficient but certainly not the only ways to apply direct pressure to the feet. Techniques can be modified for self-help. There are also many instruments which can be used safely for the care of one's feet. Generally, smooth rounded objects like golf balls or foot rollers are fine. Never, however, use any instruments on someone else's feet because it is impossible to control the pressure safely enough. This is why your thumb is such an ideal instrument. It is capable of detecting deposits, it is soft and pliable and at the same time capable of exerting varying amounts of pressure.

Choose your objectives. Target only a limited number of points for your client to work on because self-help requires a certain amount of time and dedication to the task. The objectives can always be changed but homework can be confusing and unusable if not clearly and simply defined. Carefully select a level that the subject can effectively master.

Case in Point:
One of our clients has become very enthusiastic about self help. She's been willing to try anything we suggested. Since she has an extreme allergic condition which has been a constant source of irritation and discomfort, we recommended extra homework on the adrenal areas of the hands. We told her to "pump" the adrenal reflex on each hand throughout the day and to see if it had any effect. She happily reported soon after that she was able to "turn the reactions off" by a steady pumping of her hands for three to five minutes. This gave her a sense of having some control over her condition and it pleased her greatly.

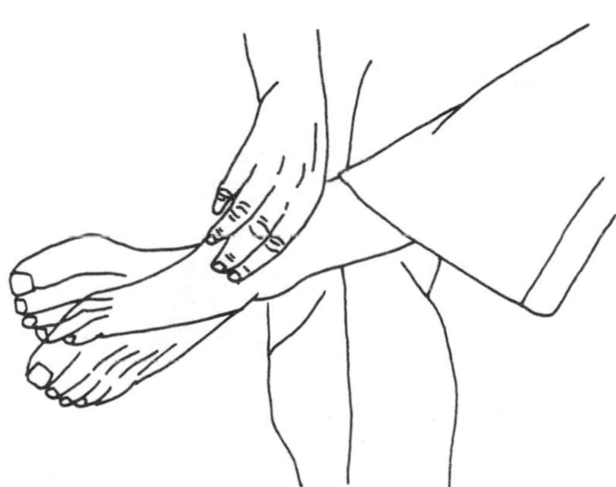

SUGGESTED TREATMENT PATTERN

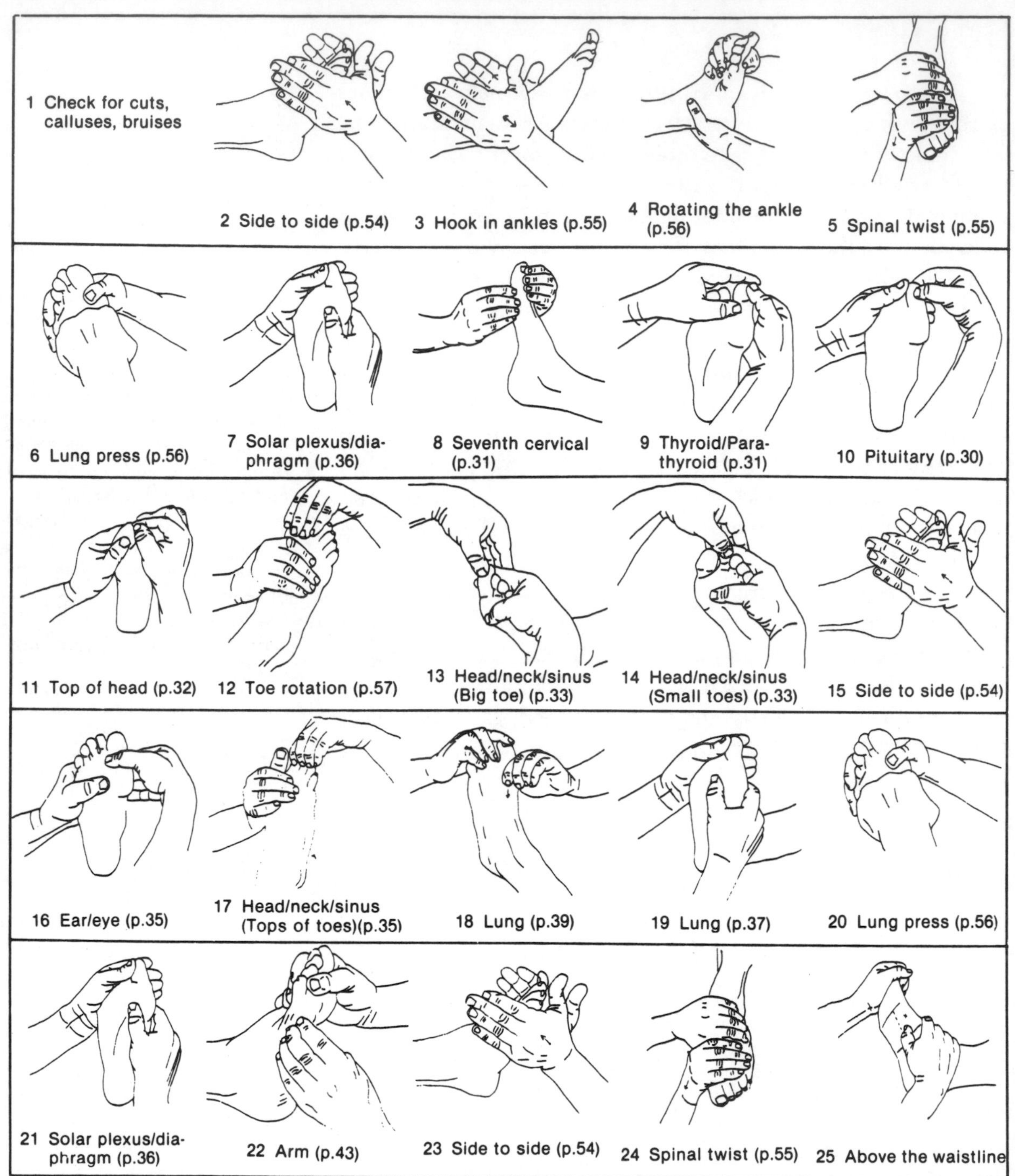
1 Check for cuts, calluses, bruises
2 Side to side (p.54)
3 Hook in ankles (p.55)
4 Rotating the ankle (p.56)
5 Spinal twist (p.55)
6 Lung press (p.56)
7 Solar plexus/dia-phragm (p.36)
8 Seventh cervical (p.31)
9 Thyroid/Para-thyroid (p.31)
10 Pituitary (p.30)
11 Top of head (p.32)
12 Toe rotation (p.57)
13 Head/neck/sinus (Big toe) (p.33)
14 Head/neck/sinus (Small toes) (p.33)
15 Side to side (p.54)
16 Ear/eye (p.35)
17 Head/neck/sinus (Tops of toes)(p.35)
18 Lung (p.39)
19 Lung (p.37)
20 Lung press (p.56)
21 Solar plexus/dia-phragm (p.36)
22 Arm (p.43)
23 Side to side (p.54)
24 Spinal twist (p.55)
25 Above the waistline

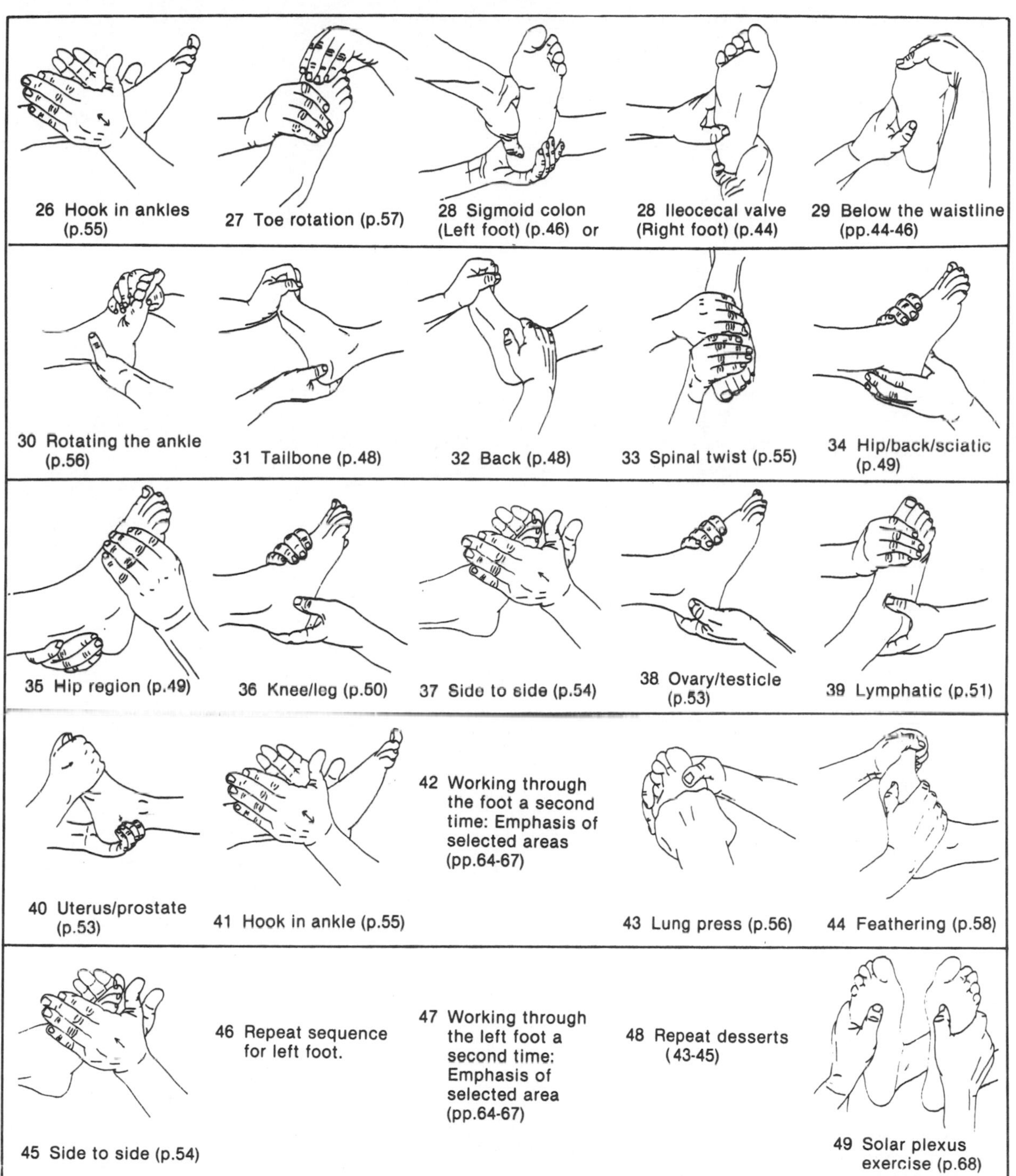
26 Hook in ankles (p.55)
27 Toe rotation (p.57)
28 Sigmoid colon (Left foot) (p.46) or
28 Ileocecal valve (Right foot) (p.44)
29 Below the waistline (pp.44-46)
30 Rotating the ankle (p.56)
31 Tailbone (p.48)
32 Back (p.48)
33 Spinal twist (p.55)
34 Hip/back/sciatic (p.49)
35 Hip region (p.49)
36 Knee/leg (p.50)
37 Side to side (p.54)
38 Ovary/testicle (p.53)
39 Lymphatic (p.51)
40 Uterus/prostate (p.53)
41 Hook in ankle (p.55)
42 Working through the foot a second time: Emphasis of selected areas (pp.64-67)
43 Lung press (p.56)
44 Feathering (p.58)
45 Side to side (p.54)
46 Repeat sequence for left foot.
47 Working through the left foot a second time: Emphasis of selected area (pp.64-67)
48 Repeat desserts (43-45)
49 Solar plexus exercise (p.68)

SUGGESTED TREATMENT PATTERN

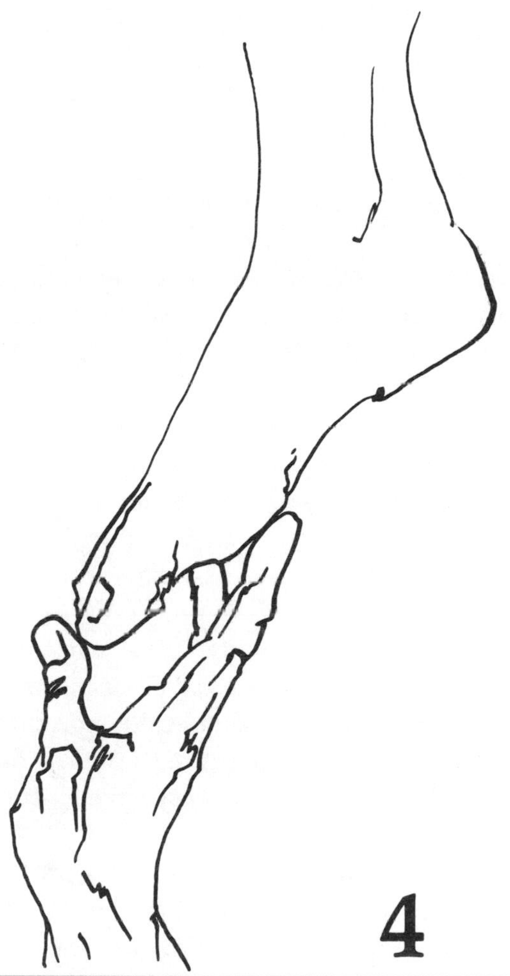

4

You the Reflexologist

YOU THE REFLEXOLOGIST

Whether you are applying reflexology as a profession or only to the feet of your family and friends, there are guidelines and rules to follow. These are essential to your professional image as a reflexologist as well as for the safety and protection of your clients and yourself. Reflexology requires a systematic approach and self discipline. Any treatment is to be taken seriously. Presenting a treatment with a well organized approach lends a great deal to your credibility.

Without a doubt, reflexology in its somewhat untraditional and revolutionary nature will continue to meet with skepticism. You will find skeptics even among family and friends. When you introduce anyone to the techniques and philosophy of reflexology, your level of confidence and self discipline in what you say and do will have a significant effect on his or her initial reaction. Obviously you cannot convert everyone but by presenting a more professional image most people will take you seriously.

In this section we will discuss the many rules and guidelines which can help you, the reflexologist. Most obviously, perhaps, you must be prepared with an accurate definition of what reflexology is and what it isn't, what it does and what it doesn't. Don't worry too much about whether your client fully understands everything you tell him. Simply offer to demonstrate. Most people do enjoy having their feet worked on. It is often a new experience for them and is most always relaxing. By offering to demonstrate, you keep a low profile and do not communicate the "hard sell" approach. Most people resent the more aggressive approach, the testimonial. How many times have you had someone tell you "This is one of the most amazing things you've ever seen! You gotta try it!" It is a temptation to tell some of the amazing health stories that are in any reflexologist's repertoire, but, let's face it, they are a bit incredible and, for many, difficult to accept. So be straightforward. Admit what you don't know. Tell your prospective client what you CAN tell, and make no promises.

Be professional. As you know, when you walk into a professional office that is appointed and managed properly, you experience the trappings of authority and stability. Authority will be communicated in subtle ways too. Your business card, the way you dress, the decor of your office should all say consistently "This reflexologist knows what he is doing." Even if you are not professionally involved in reflexology, these things are equally as important. People will regard you seriously rather than as an oddity.

The acceptance of reflexology is already changing. The image presented in newspapers is changing from a humorous one to a serious one. Remember that the evolution of the "serious" image of reflexology depends on you. For every "oddity" out there practising reflexology, it takes ten serious professionals to offset the damage done to its image.

Rules

These rules are presented in relative order of their importance. This is not to say that the last few are not important. We merely wish to place emphasis on these crucial points.

DON'T DIAGNOSE!

A foot chart is only a foot chart. There are many complex factors to consider before anyone should attempt to play doctor by diagnosing a problem based only on a basic knowledge of the reflex areas of the feet. Even though reflexology can be devastatingly accurate in giving an instant picture of a person's health condition, it can also be misinterpreted totally. Your role is *not* to find out what is wrong and diagnose it, but to apply a careful, professional combination of observation and treatment in such a way as to bring about results, *regardless of what you or your client thinks is his or her health problem.* The beauty of reflexology lies in this central fact. It works without diagnosis!

This is not to say that you cannot communicate with your client by interviewing and observation. If you are curious about soreness in a particular area of the foot, you can ask a question such as "Do you ever have trouble with your neck?" — or, "Do you ever notice difficulty moving your arm?" Don't pursue it beyond this. Take note of the answers you get. They will lead you to the areas of the feet that need extra work. Be careful not to react in such a way as to cause your client to worry about his or her health any more than he or she already is. Tell your client that soreness is very common and that it does not always indicate a chronic health problem. If your client asks you about an area, explain THAT YOU CANNOT MAKE A DIAGNOSIS. Explain the reflex areas in question and their corresponding relationship to the zones of the body. Remember that yours is the observation of a reflexologist, not the diagnosis of a medical professional.

DON'T PRESCRIBE!

One of the greatest temptations in reflexology is to combine the treatments with nutritional advice (i.e., vitamins, minerals, diets, etc.). The urge to diagnose is often followed by the urge to prescribe the instant and obvious cure. Together, these two erroneous practices can have exactly the opposite results from those you and your client are seeking. In fact, they can have disastrous results. First, you tell the person he has liver trouble, then proceed to prescribe the appropriate vitamins or diet for liver problems. If you were wrong on the first count, you're obviously wasting your time and your client's health and money on the second. Use OPINION to get your observations across. You might say something like "It might be beneficial to take more water," rather than "I recommend that you drink eight glasses of water per day." You can say something like "In my experience it is often helpful to be sure you're getting a complete, nutritional diet, with at least the minimum daily requirement of vitamins and minerals," rather than "Take two grams of vitamin C per day to correct liver deficiency." Avoid ALL TEMPTATION to prescribe ANYTHING to ANYBODY at ANYTIME! If you are asked for your opinion, give it, but be thoughtful and remember that many clients are likely to take your word as authority. Once again, tell them *only* what you *know* to be fact, and you will be going a long way toward establishing a successful and beneficial therapist-client relationship.

DON'T TREAT FOR SPECIFIC ILLNESS!

We knew of a reflexologist who regularly promised in newspaper ads to help relieve backaches and various other problems. Such advertising is, of course, asking for trouble. The written word can be powerful and often provokes the responses and actions of the authorities in medical matters. Even business cards and other forms of advertising (in the office, for example) should be carefully designed so that only an honest, straightforward approach is taken, avoiding promises to treat specific ailments and resisting the temptation to "sell" reflexology.

A reflexologist should also plan carefully just what he or she will *say* about reflexology to prospective clients. Once again it is important not to make promises to treat anything specifically. Explain that there is no way to be sure just what will be accomplished, only that you are willing to apply basic principles of reflexology to any pair of feet in a consistent and professional manner. If your client insists upon guarantees, simply state that guarantees are not a part of the program and recommend that he or she consult a physician for professional medical advice. It is better to lose a potential client than to jeopardize with legal troubles the future success and development of your work.

Finally, remember that as long as you apply the philosophy of reflexology in a professional, consistent way, striving to become ever more effective in technique and ever more observant of each pair of feet, the results will stand on their own. Prospective clients will have more faith in your low-key, confident manner when, instead of making promises you may not be able to keep, you demonstrate a well-disciplined, and consistent approach. Show them that reflexology is a system of well thought out techniques and observations whose ultimate goal is to allow every person to become involved in monitoring and maintaining his or her own health.

SO JUST WHAT DO YOU TELL YOUR CLIENT?

Now that you are aware of what NOT to do or say, let us consider what you *should* tell your client. First, learn this concise definition of reflexology:

> **Reflexology is a study of the reflexes of the feet corresponding to every part of the body. Working on these reflexes relaxes tension and helps the body to seek its own equilibrium.**

Secondly, explain the organization of the foot (use charts if possible). There should be no secrets. Be open and helpful when asked for this information. Finally, be willing to describe your techniques. Remember that part of your goal is to educate through demonstration. You should constantly encourage your clients to participate in a self help program. One way to do this is by sharing all the information you can.

GUIDELINES

As in any serious discipline, reflexology too requires hard work and dedication from those who practice it. There are no shortcuts. The fastest way to get results is the same for each pair of feet you work on: persistent application of the rules and guidelines discussed here, together with effective and efficient techniques. In each case it is the safety and comfort of your client that is at stake.

THE VISUAL OBSERVATION

Before you work any pair of feet, inspect them for abnormalities (i.e., corns, calluses, bruises, sprains, etc.) (See pages 17-19). Painful areas on the feet should be avoided. (See also "Affected Area", page 12). Note the condition of the toenails (i.e., ingrown, cracked, etc.). If severe problems exist, suggest to your client that he or she see a podiatrist.

To complete your inspection, ask your client if there are any painful or unusual conditions you should be aware of. Please note that corns and calluses should be worked. (See Table, page 108 , Giving a Treatment, page 62).

DON'T WORK AN AFFECTED AREA

Under no circumstances should you work a damaged area. If you find a cut or bruise, work around it. Similarly, if there is a foot injury (broken bone, sprain, phlebitis, etc.), do not work it but show your client corresponding areas that can be worked to benefit the injured area (See page 12).

FINGERNAIL LENGTH

The nails of the walking finger and thumb should not make contact with the skin of the foot at any time. There is, therefore, no way to have long fingernails and work safely and effectively. Proper technique simply cannot accommodate long nails because they will always cause discomfort and they may even cut the skin.

INSTRUMENTS

The beauty of reflexology lies in the safety and control achieved when applying the human hand to the human foot. In this age of advancing technology, there is a strong temptation to seek automated solutions to every working situation. Reflexologists have not been exempt from this temptation. They have tried drills, sticks, clamps, bolts, and any number of other devices to "find an easier way" to work the feet. BUT THERE IS NO EASIER WAY TO PURSUE SAFE AND EFFECTIVE TECHNIQUES THAN WITH THE HUMAN HAND. Instruments have no feeling. It is difficult to control leverage and pressure without feeling. When you lose this control, you can easily damage muscles, tendons, nerves, bones or skin. Leave instruments out of reflexology treatments.

KNUCKLES

The urge to use the knuckles to penetrate deeply into an area of the foot originates both from a misunderstanding of the principles involved and from a seeming inability to work that same area effectively with the basic techniques. While it is true that it takes time to build up your hand strength to the point where you can apply full pressure evenly for more than just a few passes, the answer is NOT the knuckles. Knuckles can cause as much damage as other instruments (See page 78). Stick to the basic finger and thumb walking techniques. Work on perfecting them and strengthening your hands so that you can vary the amount of pressure when needed and hit all the necessary points effectively and safely.

CREAMS, LOTIONS AND GOO

Creams and lotions work well for massages but not for reflexology. Lubricating the skin of the feet defeats your purpose and should not be done. While it may reduce friction between walking finger and the skin of the foot, it makes it difficult to properly hold the foot, causing loss of leverage. It also will cause you to miss many reflexes because your walking finger will slip and slide over them. You may also slip and injure a tendon or cause unnecessary discomfort. If your client wishes to use a skin cream on his or her feet after the treatment, that is fine. For perspiring feet, any mild body powder can be used.

AMOUNT OF PRESSURE

Learning how much pressure to use for different problems on different feet takes time. In the past some reflexologists measured their effectiveness by the amount of pain they could inflict. Even though we now know that some pain is inevitable and can be an excellent indicator of areas to emphasize, we have also learned that one of the primary goals of reflexology is to help the client relax. That is why the concept of a "treatment" has evolved. We use a very specific, well organized approach to working each pair of feet. Desserts (See pages 54 –59) are used at strategic times during a treatment to ease tension, to cope with stress. That's why it is so important for every reflexologist to become acutely aware of the continuity between working the reflexes and giving desserts. If the amount of pressure is too great, the client will sense that you are not in control and will begin anticipating each flood of pain. Obviously this cannot have a relaxing effect.

During a treatment work up to the tolerance point with the amount of your pressure and then back off. (Leverage is the instrument by which you can adjust the amount of pressure.) (See page 23). Above all, remember that getting results takes time. During a regular treatment program you can increase the amount of pressure you use on a client's feet as time goes on. Don't try to do it all in one treatment!!

THE LENGTH OF EACH TREATMENT

The normal amount of time for a treatment is thirty to forty-five minutes. However, if your client is ill, you should work a shorter amount of time and more often. It is not that you are endangering your client, but with full length treatments you could be making him or her more uncomfortable by putting this extra tax on his or her system.

DURATION OF PROFESSIONAL TREATMENT

It is the responsibility of the reflexologist to monitor the progress of each client from treatment to treatment. An older person with an old, chronic problem will need a great deal more time to get results than will a younger person with the same ailment. Most people begin to see some results in four to eight weeks. If the problem is more severe, it is likely to take longer. Again, consistency and regular application are the crucial factors. For a chronically ill client, it might require three treatments a week over an extended period of time. Self help application should be constantly encouraged (See page 69).

FREQUENCY OF TREATMENT

Under normal circumstances, start your client out at twice a week. In some cases you may want it to be even more frequent than that. Since the key to results through reflexology is regular application, two times per week ensures that your client will have a full treatment about every three days. Combined with self help (See page 69) this arrangement will bring optimum results.

During the course of the treatments, as improvements are noted and the client's feet become normalized, reduce the frequency of treatments as desired.

REACTIONS

Occasionally after a treatment your client may have some kind of reaction. Normally this will be a general feeling of discomfort throughout the body, and sometimes there is even a temporary feeling of illness. Don't panic if this happens. Reassure your client by explaining that this is common and should pass quickly. If there is a problem that seems to be a reaction at first but continues, it may not be a reaction and you should suggest that your client seek medical help.

Since most reactions are caused by the sudden release of toxins or waste products into the system, one way of avoiding them is by working the kidney area thoroughly on each foot (See page 44) during the first several treatments with a new client. Even the most healthy looking people can have these temporary reactions.

POSITIONING, POSTURE AND EYE CONTACT

Your client's feet should be elevated enough so that your arms and back are not unduly strained. A recliner with extending foot rest is an excellent way to ensure your client's comfort and to get the feet up high enough for you to work on. Sit on a low stool or small chair so that your client's feet are at about your chest level. In this position you can also keep an eye on your client's facial expressions, allowing you to know when you are reaching the tolerance level with the amount of your pressure (See page 79). Each person is unique, and direct eye contact from this posture enables you to study and become acquainted with each person's way of reacting to your treatment. If your client is lying prone for any reason during the treatment (illness, paralysis, or in conjunction with another therapy), be sure the head is propped slightly on a pillow so that you can maintain the eye contact. Otherwise you could be causing your client pain and not realize it.

WORKING ON BARE FEET If at all possible work on bare feet. Nylons or stockings get in the way and are hard on the walking fingers. Some clients may not expect this so always explain it before the first treatment.

WASHING YOUR HANDS Always wash your hands after working on a pair of feet. Make it a habit. It not only makes sense hygenically but it will contribute to your professional image. Cleanliness is a part of thoroughness.

GENERAL ISSUES

MYTHS

There are more myths about reflexology than there are pages in this book. They can have harmful effects because, just like rumors, they always seem to have a willing audience. Let's look at a few of the worst ones.

Myth: REFLEXOLOGY IS NOT SAFE FOR BABIES

Fact: Not true. Reflexology is safe for EVERYONE! In fact, children love to have their feet worked on because they can experience the immediate and natural pleasure of it. Light pressure is used on the feet of infants, and has even been known to relieve colic. The techniques must be adapted to tiny feet. In general, babies enjoy and benefit from very light pressure on the bottoms of their feet.

Myth: REFLEXOLOGY IS NOT SAFE FOR PREGNANT WOMEN

Fact: Not true. If the fear is of miscarriage, reflexology can only *help* the body seek its own equilibrium. A miscarriage is a reaction of the body, NOT a reaction to reflexology. Under no circumstances has reflexology ever been shown to have caused the body to do something it didn't want to do.

Myth: REFLEXOLOGY IS NOT SAFE FOR DIABETICS

Fact: Not true. Insulin shock is the result of the improper treatment of diabetes. It is NOT the result of, nor does it have any connection with reflexology treatments. A person who is diabetic has a serious health problem which requires constant attention. Reflexology can and should be used with diabetics as well as with any ill persons to help restore homeostasis.

REFLEXOLOGY CAN CAUSE HEART ATTACKS *Myth*

Fact Not true. A young reflexologist once told us that she had "given a man a heart attack." Upon investigation we learned that she had given the man one reflexology treatment the week before his heart attack. She thought she had caused it! It is often possible to detect buildup and tenderness in the chest area on the feet of a person with heart trouble. But it is not possible to diagnose heart trouble based on such condition of the feet. Suggest that if he or she feels anything unusual they should consult a physician immediately.

IS REFLEXOLOGY SAFE?

Reflexology is in itself totally safe. With restraint and common sense a reflexologist can keep it that way. Since there is some pain involved in the elimination of buildup in the reflex areas, it should be used as a signal to prevent working too fast or too hard. If you find a reflexologist who insists on using pressure past the point of your tolerance, tell him or her that this is improper and find another reflexologist if necessary.

There is a tendon which runs down the bottom of each foot that is of particular concern. (See page 40) Never work the tendon while it is pulled taut. A slight release of the hold on the toes will prevent bruising and possibly damaging it.

ETHICS AND PROFESSIONALISM

You probably noticed that the subject of your professionalism has been touched upon several times in this chapter. Whether you are a full time professional reflexologist or not, strive always to present a good image to your client or to the relative or friend whose feet you are working on.

The enjoyment and rewards of reflexology are by-products of your ability to help individuals. Accepting your role as reflexologist requires the understanding that you have a responsibility to the person you are working on. It demands a great deal of personal self discipline and the desire to help others.

Once you've learned the techniques, your real responsibilities begin. There are three important components: professional attitude, ethical business conduct and a continuing self education program.

Your attitudes are important. Do YOU take your work seriously? Can you accept the fact that it is better not to boast of your accomplishments and the accomplishments of reflexology? Do you exude a quiet confidence in what you do, without taking the "hard sell" approach? Can you define what you do and explain concisely and accurately all of the concepts?

Ethical business conduct is, of course, important to each of us. Continuing education as in all professional endeavors, demonstrate to the client that you are constantly exploring and updating your practice, that you are interested in providing the best service possible. Continuing self education includes study in reflexology and related fields, such as anatomy.

As in any profession it is essential that a practitioner make a constant effort to keep up to date on new concepts and advances in the field. In reflexology, start with a variety of anatomy books and a good medical dictionary. Update yourself through exposure to current writing on reflexology.[1]

CONTINUING SELF EDUCATION

PROMOTING YOUR BUSINESS

The best advertising you can have is satisfied clientele. Good results from safe and competent application of reflexology coupled with sound professionalism in the office will spread the word loudly and clearly. You will find that most of your new clients will have been referred to you by your other clients.

Even if you follow all the rules and practice in a professional and safe manner, you may yet have legal problems. Reflexology has not yet come into full acceptance. Ignorance

[1] An excellent example is **REFLEXIONS©**, a periodic newsletter devoted exclusively to current issues and developments in reflexology. Available from Reflexology Research Project, 6209 Hendrix NE, Albuquerque, N.M. 87110.

and misunderstanding in your community can hurt you. Make a continuing effort to clarify what reflexology is and what it does. Don't boast of your accomplishments. Let your clients do that. It is, after all, their bodies which have done the healing! But if reason and moderation don't work and you are being harassed either privately or officially, seek the help of a lawyer. One reflexologist in Illinois was effective dealing with various state agencies with the aid of her lawyer.

PROFESSIONALISM

A well organized office gives credibility to the professional reflexologist. In general, a conservative approach suits the health field. This applies to your dress, interior decorating and all promotional material. Neat, clean business attire, regular office furniture and a well laid out business card will present a stable image to potential clients. Let's face it. Reflexology is unique and somewhat unusual. A person entering your office for the first time is uncertain about you and maybe about reflexology too. He will be looking for signs of stability and will relate to an environment with which he is likely to be familiar. This doesn't mean that your office must be straightlaced. There is room for creativity and for humor.

BUSINESS ETHICS

Be ethical in all your dealings. Professional business practices are necessary to avoid serious repercussions that hurt not only you and your reputation but that of reflexology as well. Read and reread the rules and guidelines on pages 75 to 82 of this chapter.

You should always be straightforward about fees, scheduling procedures, hours, and other information that could prevent misunderstandings later on. Provide clear ground rules about missed appointments, lateness, and anything else that could disrupt the smooth operation of your business.

Depending upon the laws in your area, it might be a good idea to prepare a card clearly stating what you *don't* do (See Illus. page 86). Have each client read and sign it to certify their understanding of the arrangement. This can be very important because many people may have expectations about your "medical" abilities before they actually find out what reflexology is all about.

We are not doctors.
We will not diagnose, prescribe for, or treat any specific illness. If you have a medical problem, we urge you to seek professional medical help.
We are working on

____

at his/her request.
I have read and understand the above.

Signed______________________________

Date ______________________________

LICENSING

At the time of this writing there exists no official licensing for reflexologists in the United States. Requirements for legality vary greatly from jurisdiction to jurisdiction.

We have discussed the general guidelines and have developed rules pertaining to safe treatment and professional practice. Perhaps guidelines such as these will be a part of the licensing procedures for reflexologists in the future.

Licensing is an inevitable governmental control for reflexology as it evolves into a common profession. But it is not a simple matter. The concept of the licensed practice of reflexology cannot be allowed to inhibit individuals from providing their own self help program. Just as barbers are licensed to charge fees for cutting hair while individuals are free to cut their own, *so must reflexologists prepare for the day when standards will be set and licenses issued, even though they will continue to be free to work on the feet of family and friends.* Until that time all persons involved in the practice of reflexology must share the responsibility for its reputation and growth. For now, self regulation and common sense, as outlined in this chapter, can help keep the growth of reflexology a positive one.

Finally, don't think of or treat the medical professional as your enemy. Approach the medical community with the attitude that your work is complementary to, rather than a replacement for, theirs.

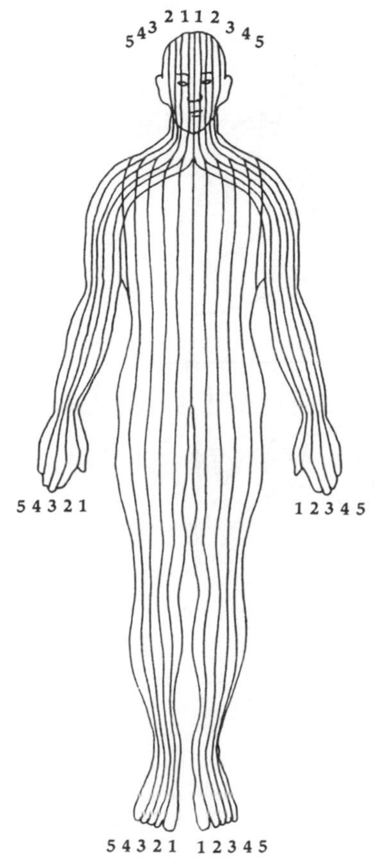
5 4 3 2 1 1 2 3 4 5
5 4 3 2 1
1 2 3 4 5
5 4 3 2 1 1 2 3 4 5

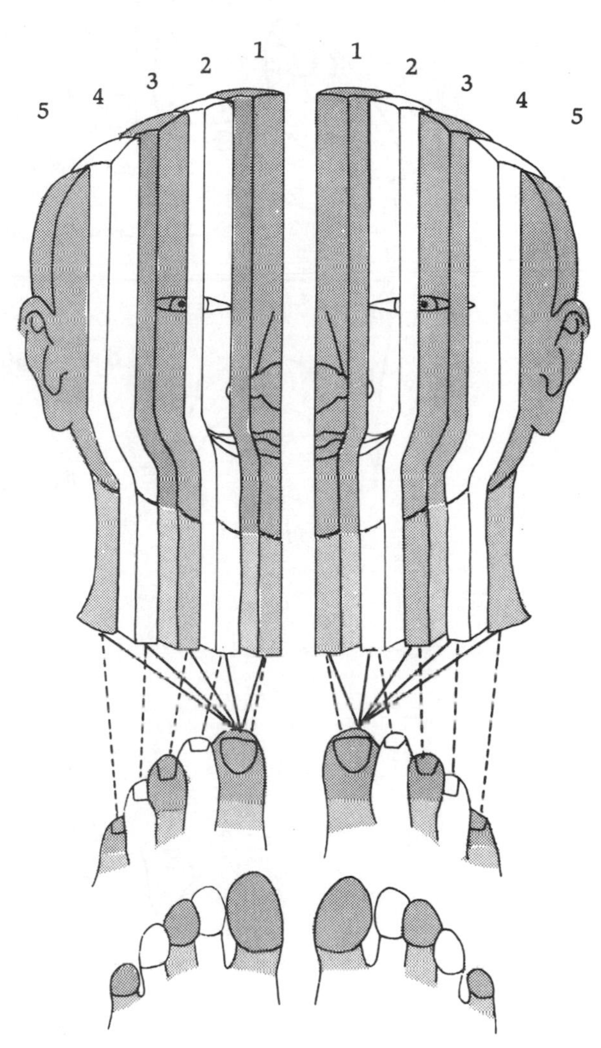
5 4 3 2 1
1 2 3 4 5

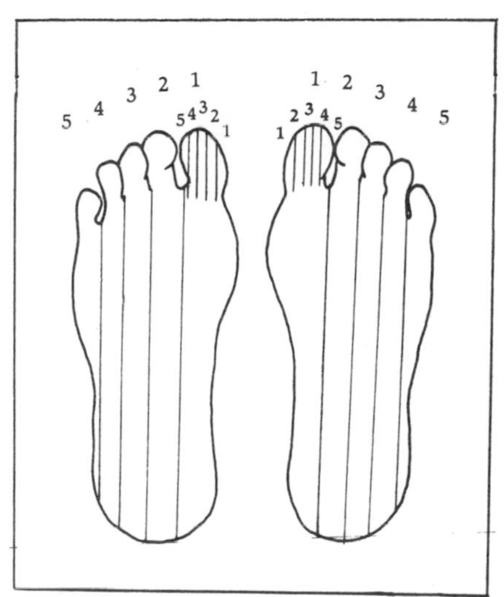
5 4 3 2 1
5 4 3 2 1
1 2 3 4 5
1 2 3 4 5

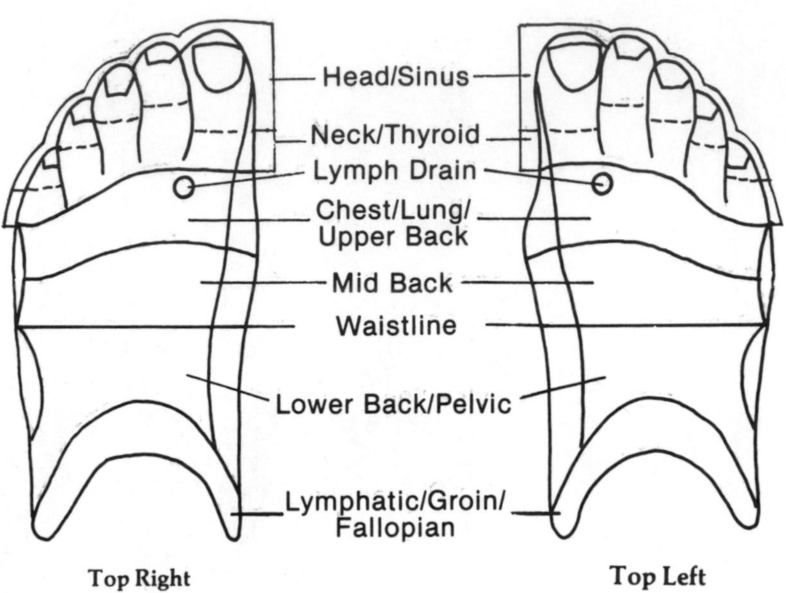
Head/Sinus
Neck/Thyroid
Lymph Drain
Chest/Lung/
Upper Back
Mid Back
Waistline
Lower Back/Pelvic
Lymphatic/Groin/
Fallopian
Top Right
Top Left

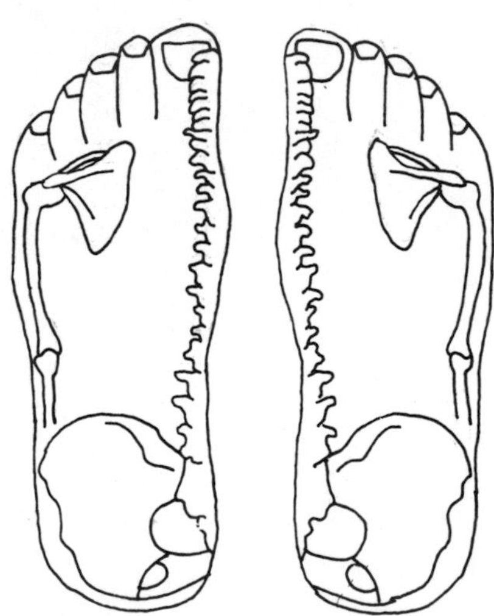

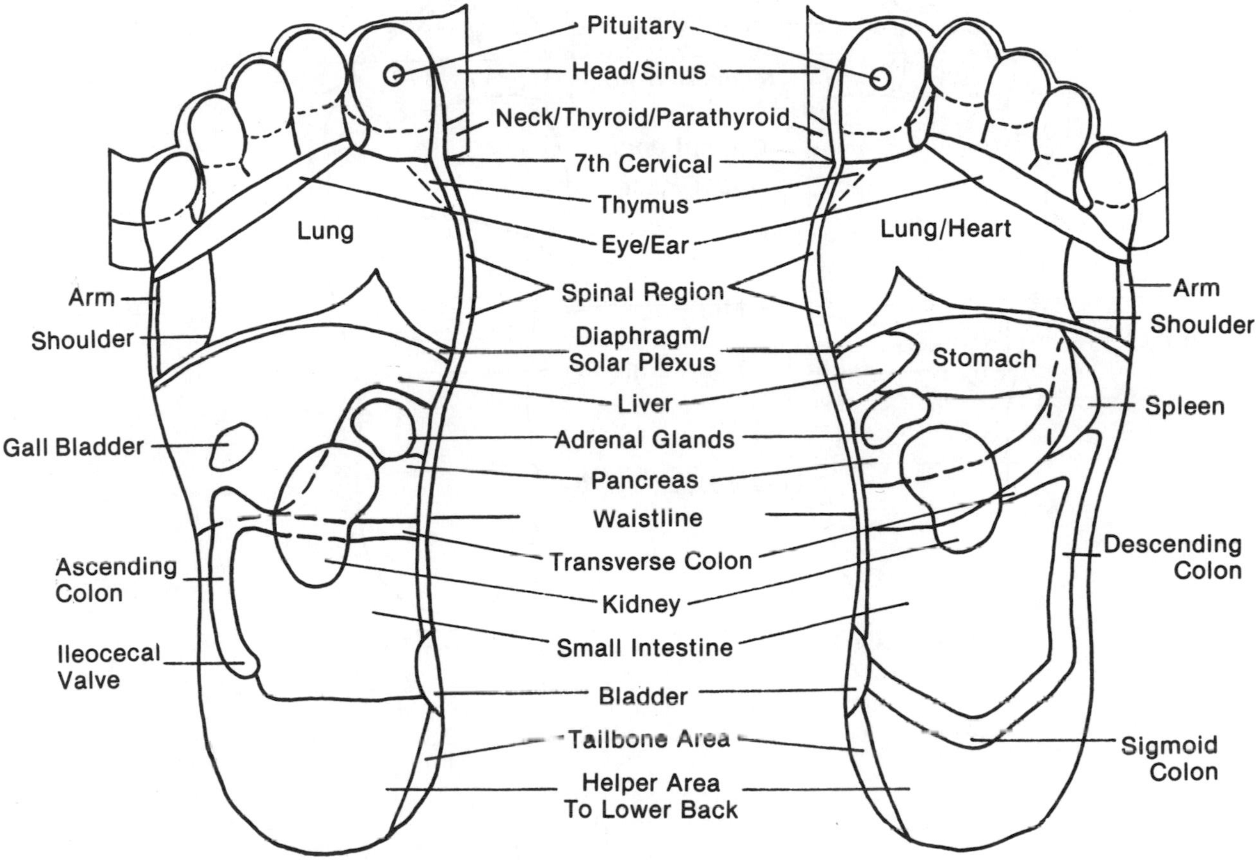

Pituitary
Head/Sinus
Neck/Thyroid/Parathyroid
7th Cervical
Thymus
Lung
Lung/Heart
Eye/Ear
Arm
Spinal Region
Arm
Shoulder
Diaphragm/
Solar Plexus
Shoulder
Stomach
Liver
Spleen
Gall Bladder
Adrenal Glands
Pancreas
Waistline
Descending
Colon
Ascending
Colon
Transverse Colon
Kidney
Ileocecal
Valve
Small Intestine
Bladder
Tailbone Area
Sigmoid
Colon
Helper Area
To Lower Back

Bottom Right

Bottom Left

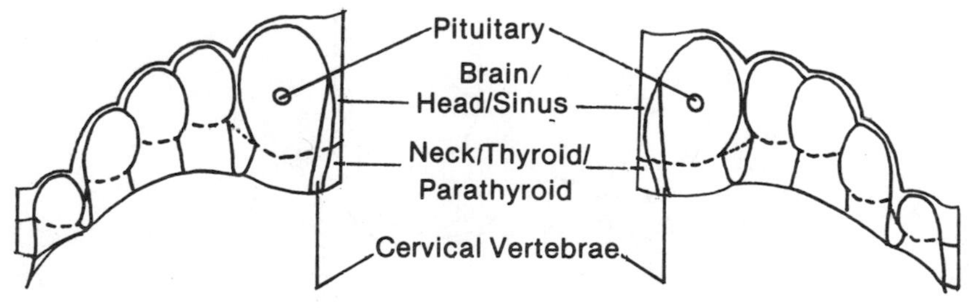

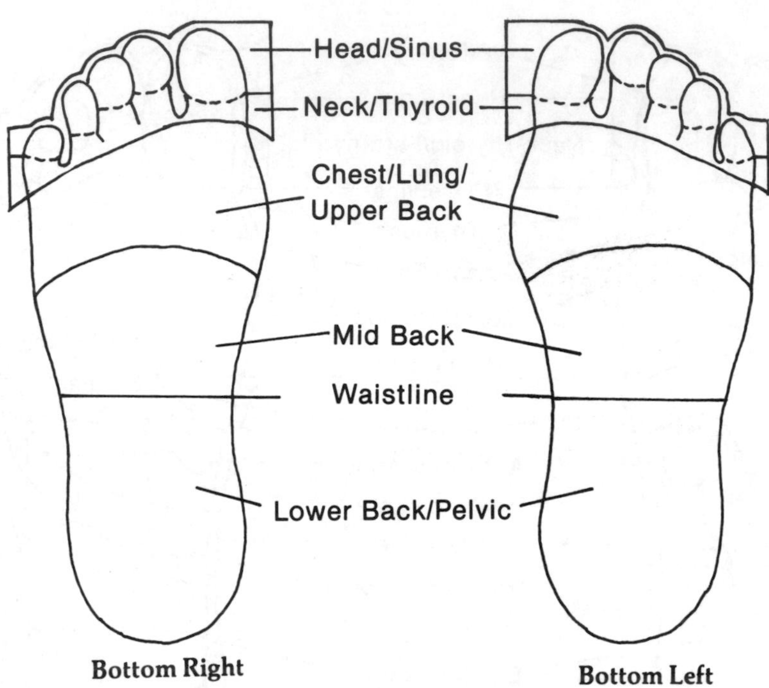
Head/Sinus
Neck/Thyroid
Chest/Lung/
Upper Back
Mid Back
Waistline
Lower Back/Pelvic
Bottom Right
Bottom Left

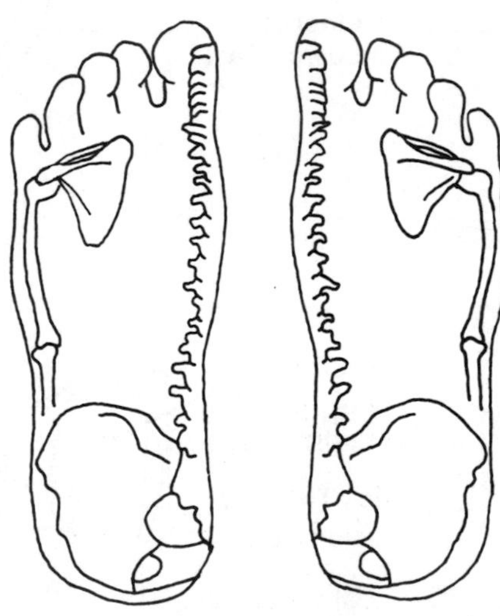

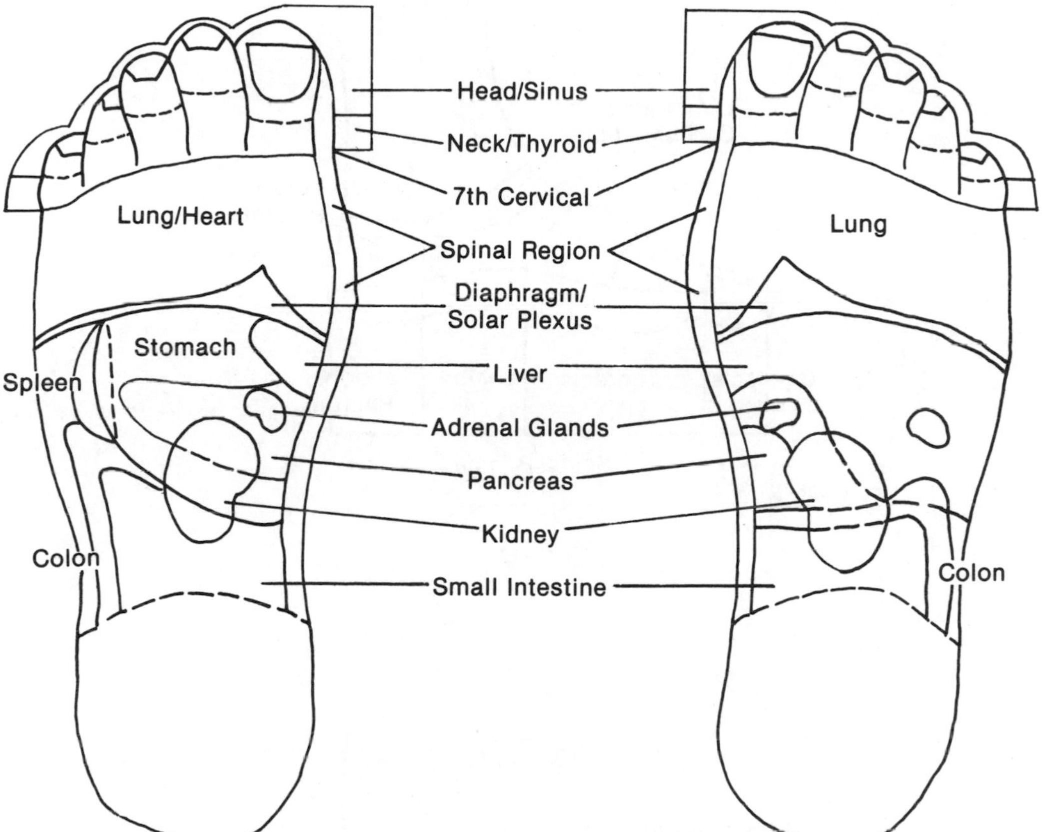

Head/Sinus
Neck/Thyroid
7th Cervical
Lung/Heart
Lung
Spinal Region
Diaphragm/
Solar Plexus
Stomach
Spleen
Liver
Adrenal Glands
Pancreas
Kidney
Colon
Colon
Small Intestine

Top Left

Top Right

Brain /
Head/Sinus
Neck/Thyroid/
Parathyroid
Cervical
Vertebrae

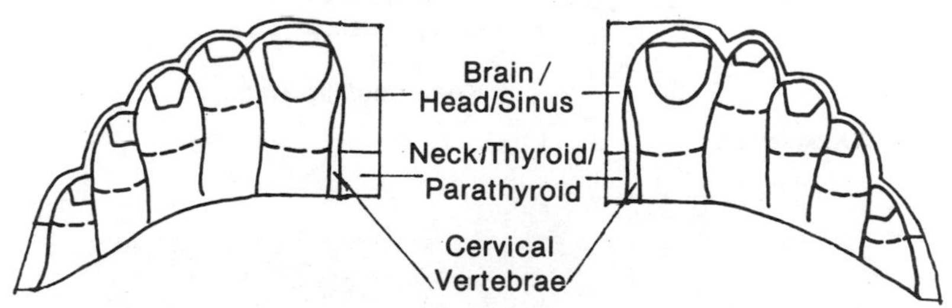

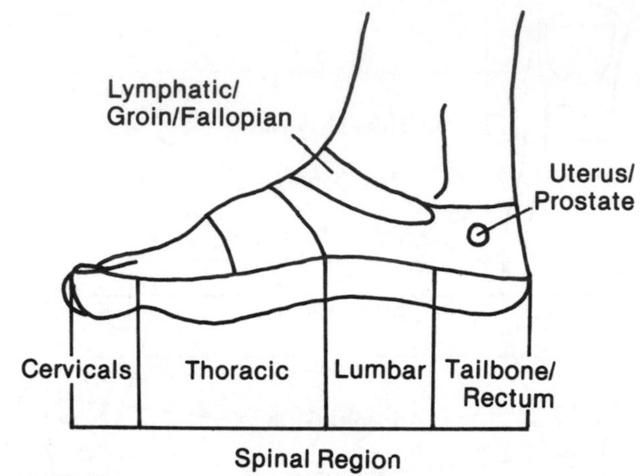

Inside Right

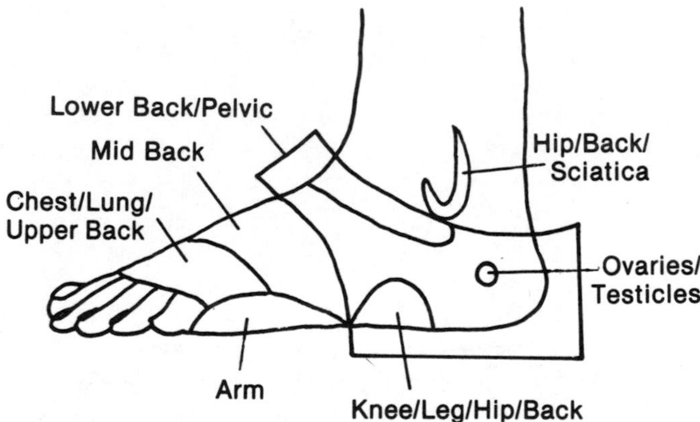

Outside Left

The Complete Guide to Foot Reflexology

DISORDER	QUICK REFERENCE	
Infertility		
Male	Testes (pp.52-53) Prostate (pp.52-53)	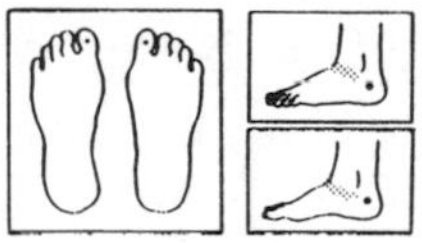
Female	Uterus (pp.52-53) Ovaries (pp.52-53) Fallopian Tubes (p. 51) Pituitary (p. 30)	
Kidney Disorders	Kidney (pp.40-42,44) Ureter Tubes (p. 45) Bladder (pp.47-48) Adrenal Glands (with infection) (pp.40-42)	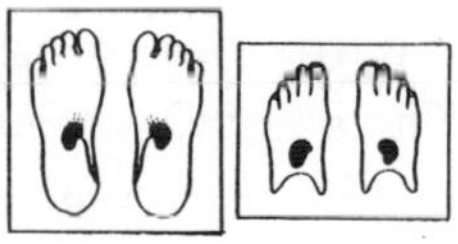
Kidney Stones	Kidneys (pp.40-42,44) Ureter Tubes (p. 45) Bladder (pp.47-48)	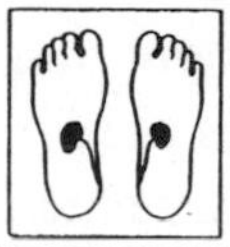
Lower Back *See*	*Back* *Hip Disorders* *Sciatica*	

5

Anatomy

Table of Disorders

Anatomy

Table of Disorders

It is the basic premise of reflexology that maintaining the human body is a complex problem which can be simplified by understanding how every part of the body is related to areas on the feet. That constipation, for example, can be reflected in the lower back reflex area of the feet suggests that the more one knows about the anatomy of the abdominal-pelvic region of the body, the more efficient and precise will be the understanding and treatment of problems in that area of the body. This is true, of course, for the whole body. A working knowledge of anatomy is essential to understanding the organizational scheme of the feet. Since health problems are not simple and are seldom isolated to one organ or part of the body, a reflexologist familiar with basic anatomy can approach any problem more efficiently by working several areas in conjunction with each other.

This chapter has two sections: **Anatomy** and **Table of Symptoms and Disorders.** The first is a discussion of anatomical function with brief comments on some important symptoms or disorders regulated by that organ or part. The second is an alphabetical table of symptoms or disorders with suggestions for areas of the feet to emphasize with reflexology. The two sections interrelate and can be used together to help the reflexologist give controlled emphasis to problem areas during treatments.

The need for learning basic anatomy does not in any way detract from a reflexologist's ability to treat the body as a whole. Decisions as to which areas on the feet to emphasize DO NOT depend on medical diagnosis. It is very easy to succumb to the temptation to make a quick diagnosis based on a little knowledge of anatomy, but a reflexologist should remember that the roots of reflexology lie in zone theory. The zone theory system is holistic, that is, it integrates the body into a whole and, instead of giving specific, concrete answers through diagnosis, it simply points the way for the thumbs and fingers of the reflexologist.

Reflexology has been used successfully in the treatment of all of the symptoms and disorders discussed in this chapter. There have been and will be varying degrees of success related to a number of factors (i.e., how old is the problem, how frequent are the treatments, how effective are the techniques, etc.). There can be no doubt that together the refinement of technique and basic knowledge of anatomy form an imposing partnership which can only enhance this success rate.

ENDOCRINE SYSTEM

Pituitary
Adrenal
Thyroid
Parathyroid
Pancreas
Reproductive

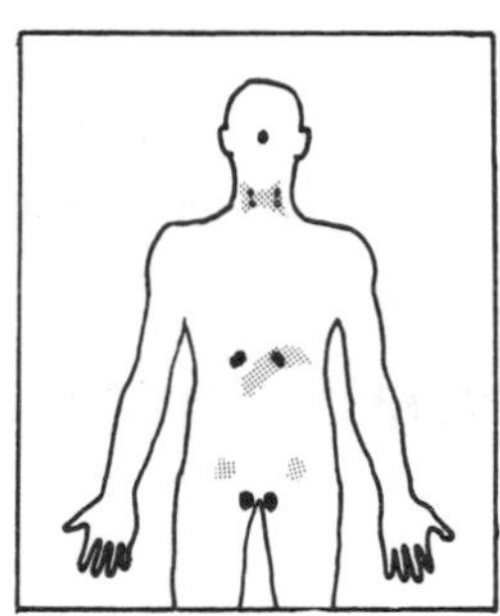

The endocrine glands serve as regulators. Together with the central nervous system they are responsible for controlling the complex activities of the body. Their messengers, the hormones, transmit their messages all over the body. There are many hormones serving many functions.

The endocrine glands are ductless, secreting their hormones directly into the blood stream. These glands can malfunction either by being overactive (hyperactive) or underactive (hypoactive). Serious malfunction can result in such disorders as tetany, Addison's Disease, diabetes and dwarfism. Less critical malfunctions may result in subtle changes in the metabolism, physical and sexual development, mental well-being and overall body health.

As the reflexologist relieves stress (the source of many of these problems) the body is allowed to seek its own hormonal equilibrium.

PITUITARY

Think of the endocrine glands as a large management team. Its chief executive would be the pituitary. The pituitary gland is located at the base of the brain and is approximately one-half inch in diameter. It produces a number of hormones performing many different functions.

PITUITARY FUNCTIONS

growth

Effects hard and soft tissue growth. "Growth" can be defined as structural growth (such as body height). An imbalance in the pituitary can produce giantism or dwarfism. "Growth" can also be of soft tissue (such as tumors). The pituitary is involved in any type of growth, normal or abnormal.

metabolism Metabolism is the rate at which cells work. The pituitary is the chief regulator, supervising the other glands involved in this process.

regulation The pituitary regulates the other endocrine glands, the arteries of the heart and body, water balance, blood pressure, sexual maturation and reproduction.

DYSFUNCTIONS CONTROLLED BY THE PITUITARY GLAND

fever Fever is a type of defensive reaction to protect the body. If the temperature of the body gets too high, its well-being is jeopardized. Together with the hypothalamus, the pituitary is involved in the body's attempt to cope with fever. (See Table pg. 124)

fainting The pituitary secretes a hormone called vasopressin, which regulates arterial constriction. Since fainting results from a sudden insufficient blood supply to the brain, this hormone, and thus the pituitary, are involved.

THYROID GLAND

The thyroid gland regulates the basal metabolism of the body cells. It is located in the front of the neck and is "H-shaped".

THYROID FUNCTIONS

metabolism Metabolism refers to the rate at which the body uses absorbed foods. It burns them to get heat and energy for its activities. Extreme overactivity or underactivity causes obvious physical changes in weight, as well as in physical and mental acuity. The thyroid produces thyroxin, a hormone which increases the rates of activity of almost all of the chemical reactions in all the cells of the body.

growth and development The thyroid produces a hormone which effects bone growth. It also controls calcium levels with calcitonin, a hormone which facilitates the movement of calcium into the bone. This operates in opposition to the parathyroid hormone which increases the movement of calcium from the bone into the blood. The effect of the growth hormone of the pituitary gland is insignificant without the presence of thyroxin.

DYSFUNCTIONS CONTROLLED BY THE THYROID GLANDS

The thyroid asserts control over skin health. An underactive thyroid can result in dryness of skin. The outer layer of the skin is a covering of dry, dead cells that are constantly being shed and replaced by cells from the growing layer. If the rate at which the cells are being disposed of is abnormal, dryness of skin results. A deficiency of thyroid function directly controls this rate.

dryness of skin

The thyroid does have an effect on the cholesterol level in the body. Cholesterol is a fat-like substance found in most tissues and is a main component of the lining of the arteries. If the level of cholesterol is too high, it can contribute to arteriosclerosis, or hardening of the arteries.

cholesterol

PARATHYROID GLANDS

The parathyroids are imbedded in the thyroid. Their hormone controls the levels of calcium and phosphorous in the blood. The level of calcium in the blood is important because it is involved in blood clotting, contraction of muscles, and the actions of the nerves. Most of the phosphorus in the body is combined with calcium in the bone, and the balance of assimilation and excretion of phosphorous is closely linked to that of calcium.

PARATHYROID FUNCTIONS

Bone is constantly being broken down and renewed. The parathyroid's job is to take calcium from this "reservoir" and add it to the body fluids when needed. The concentration of calcium in the body fluids can do its job properly only if kept within very narrow limits.

calcium levels

DYSFUNCTIONS CONTROLLED BY THE PARATHYROID

Calcium and phosphorous are essential to the normal operation of the muscles and nerves. Parathyroid failure often causes an imbalance in calcium and phosphorous levels, which can result in muscle contractions, the serious form of which is called tetany.

cramps

ADRENAL GLANDS

The adrenal glands are located on top of the kidneys. They have some fifty functions that interrelate with the other glands and are regulated by the pituitary.

ADRENAL FUNCTIONS

adrenalin production

Adrenalin is the "fight or flight" hormone. It stimulates heart action, releases glucose, raises the blood pressure and increases the circulation of the blood to the muscles. It relaxes air passages, stimulates breathing and prepares the body for action. In order to do this it must slow down digestive and excretive processes, reducing the blood flow to all areas except the muscles and heart.

muscle operation

The arterial, heart and digestive muscles are involuntary in nature. The adrenal glands secrete hormones which have an effect on these muscles. For instance, peristalsis (wave-like contractions in the intestines) is necessary to propel the food along the digestive tract. The adrenal glands must maintain the muscle tone in the digestive tract to promote normal, healthy peristalsis.

water and mineral balance

The adrenals secrete hormones which control the water and mineral balances, which in turn effect the operations of the muscles.

DYSFUNCTIONS CONTROLLED BY THE ADRENAL GLANDS

inflammation

Inflammation is a natural result of the body's attempt to heal itself. The adrenal glands produce a natural form of cortisone which aids in reducing inflammation. An injection of synthetic cortisone tends to signal the adrenal glands that enough cortisone is in the system. Prolonged use of synthetic cortisone can thus have serious side effects. Chief among them is inhibiting the natural function of the glands themselves.

stress

The adrenal glands help the body to combat stress. Cortisone prevents stress from becoming lethal to living tissue. Cortical hormones and adrenalin are main elements in the body's fight against fatigue. Fatigue lowers the body's ability to handle stress. (Stress is defined as injury, infection, environmental factors, psychological strain, etc.)

asthma

Because of the ability of adrenalin to open air passages, it is often administered in the treatment of asthma.

arthritis

Cortisone (see "Inflammation" pg. 94) is commonly used by the body to fight the inflammation associated with arthritis.

allergy

An allergic reaction is the body's response to the presence of certain types of food, clothing or other physical matter in the body's immediate environment. Adrenalin and cortisone are two of the body's natural weapons against allergies.

low blood pressure

Blood pressure is the force exerted by the heart in pumping blood from its chambers. It is affected by the amount of adrenalin and noradrenalin produced by the adrenal glands. Adrenalin permits emergency contraction of some parts of the body and emergency relaxation of others. Noradrenalin is involved with contraction primarily and thus handles such jobs as the maintenance of proper blood pressure. Thus noradrenalin has an effect on long term stress.

PANCREAS

The pancreas lies mainly behind the stomach across the back of the abdomen. It is a dual-purpose organ with endocrine function (ductless: hormones are secreted directly into the blood stream) and exocrine function (ducted: digestive juices are secreted through the pancreatic duct).

PANCREAS FUNCTIONS

digestion (exocrine)

Pancreatic juice is alkaline and neutralizes acid from the stomach. It has many enzymes which are catalysts that break down complex substances into simpler substances for absorption through the intestine into the blood stream.

blood sugar level (endocrine)

Insulin, a hormone produced by the pancreas is essential in controlling the glucose level in the blood. Glucose is the principal energy food used by the body.

DYSFUNCTIONS CONTROLLED BY THE PANCREAS

diabetes

Diabetes is a condition in which the pancreas fails to supply enough insulin to control the blood sugar (glucose) levels. There are many serious side effects and, unless sufficient insulin is supplied, diabetes can be fatal. The eyes and kidneys are usually the first to be affected if diabetes is not treated. This condition can occur during childhood as well as later in life. Juvenile diabetes is the more difficult and the more serious. Injections of insulin (or oral administration) and strict control of diet are common forms of treatment.

hypoglycemia

Hypoglycemia is a condition in which the pancreas produces too much insulin, thereby creating a low blood sugar level. Many symptoms accompany a low blood sugar condition. For example, the brain has no fuel reserve except the supply of glucose in the blood. Hypoglycemia will impair the efficiency of the brain. It is principally through the regulation of diet that hypoglycemia is commonly treated.

REPRODUCTIVE GLANDS

All body cells require hormones just as all cells require nutrients. Virtually every cell in the body is affected by the hormones produced by the reproductive organs. The importance of the role these hormones play is felt throughout the human life cycle.

FUNCTIONS OF THE REPRODUCTIVE ORGANS

sex hormones

Sex hormones influence the reproductive capacities, maintain sexual urge, and influence mental vigor and physical development.

DYSFUNCTIONS CONTROLLED BY THE REPRODUCTIVE ORGANS

allergies

The reproductive organs produce hormones used by the adrenal glands and vice versa. This relationship may account for the effect the reproductive organs have in helping the body cope with allergies.

infertility

Dysfunction of the reproductive organs (i.e., low sperm count, blocked fallopian tube, irregular ovulation, suppressed sexual urge, etc.) results in the inability to conceive a child.

Digestive system

Stomach
Liver
Gallbladder
Small Intestine
Ileocecal Valve
Large Intestine

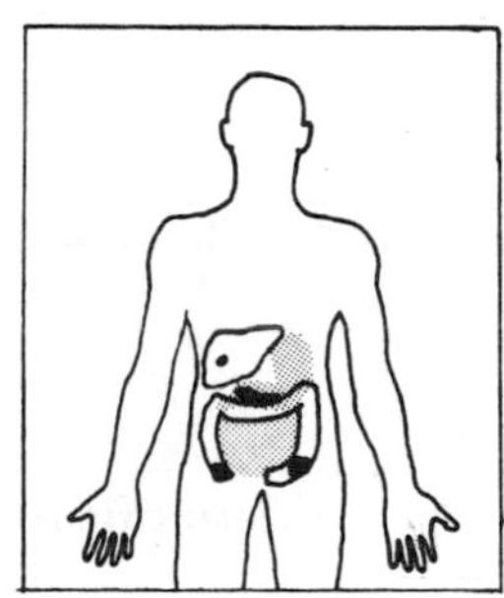

The digestive system takes the complex molecules of our food and breaks them down into simpler forms that are essential for the body's operations.

The process starts with ingestion and ends with the disposal of the waste from the system. The digestive system is actually a long tube with various secretions from different organs being added along the way.

The major organs considered here are the stomach, liver, gallbladder, pancreas, large and small intestines.

STOMACH

The stomach is that part of the digestive tract located between the esophagus (food pipe) and the duodenum, the first portion of the small intestine. It is dilated and sac-like in shape. The stomach is a neutral organ. Most of its common problems originate elsewhere.

STOMACH FUNCTIONS

digestion

During its two or three hour stay in the stomach, food is processed into a thin mash. With the exception of substances such as water and alcohol, no absorption of food takes place here. When food enters the stomach the hormone gastrin is released into the blood to stimulate the secretion of gastric acids.

DYSFUNCTIONS CONTROLLED BY THE STOMACH

ulcer

A stomach ulcer is an open sore on the mucus membrane lining of the stomach. Emotional stress can promote the secretion of acid and is almost certainly a cause of stomach ulcers. Also, certain types of physical stress (e.g. extensive burns) can have the same effect.

LIVER

The liver is the body's largest gland. It occupies the upper right and part of the upper left side of the abdominal cavity. It is essential to life.

LIVER FUNCTIONS

detoxification

Poisoning of the liver is common because anything absorbed from the stomach is carried first to the liver for detoxification. The liver, therefore, gets a higher concentration of poisons than other organs. Many drugs and industrial chemicals can damage the liver during its attempt to protect the rest of the body. Alcohol is the most common of the poisons which the liver seeks to neutralize.

digestion

During digestion the liver retains glycogen, a storable form of glucose, which enables it to supply a steady concentration to the blood, replacing what has been consumed as fuel. The brain keeps no stores at all and quickly dies if the supplies from the liver are cut off. It also stores proteins, fats, minerals and vitamins for later use.

bile

Bile is a secretion of the liver which helps break down the proteins, carbohydrates, and particularly the fats to prepare them for absorption into the blood system. Bile also lubricates the digestive tract.

GALLBLADDER

The gallbladder is imbedded in the liver. It acts as a storehouse for the bile, releasing it as needed.

GALLBLADDER FUNCTIONS

bile storage

Bile accumulates in the gallbladder until after a heavy meal. Fats stimulate the secretion of the bile. Its active functions depend on bile salts formed in the liver from cholesterol. This emulsifies the fat, making it easy to digest.

DYSFUNCTIONS CONTROLLED BY THE GALLBLADDER

gallstones

Fat particles, particularly cholesterol, can crystallize from the bile forming gallstones in the gallbladder.

SMALL INTESTINES

The beginning of the small intestine is the "C shaped" duodenum where the digestion of food is brought near completion. The remainder of the small intestine is a long, narrow tube (22.5 ft.) lined with a vast number of small, fingerlike projections called villi, which absorb the nutrients from the digested food.

SMALL INTESTINE FUNCTIONS

peristalsis

Peristalsis is the wavelike contraction of the muscles of the intestines which propels the food along the digestive tract.

absorption

Nutrients are absorbed by the villi of the small intestines and then "pumped" out to the blood and lymph vessels leading from the villi.

ILEOCECAL VALVE

The ileocecal valve is a passageway between the small and large intestine. Its principal function is to prevent backflow of fecal contents from the colon into the small intestine.

DYSFUNCTIONS CONTROLLED BY THE ILEOCECAL VALVE

mucus control

Mucus is a clear fluid forming a protective barrier on the surfaces of the lining of membranes. The area around the ileocecal valve is responsible for the control of mucus. If the mucus is not controlled properly it can break up and be absorbed into the digestive system. Mucus control is important in related problems such as sinus problems and lung problems.

LARGE INTESTINES

The large intestine is much wider than the small intestine and about five feet long. It consists of the ascending, transverse, and descending colon (including sigmoid and rectum).

LARGE INTESTINE FUNCTIONS

absorption

The colon absorbs water and electrolytes from the waste material.

storage

The colon stores fecal matter until it can be expelled.

URINARY SYSTEM

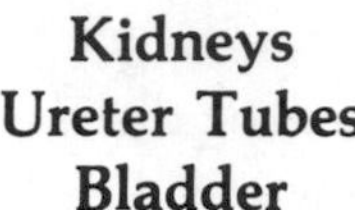

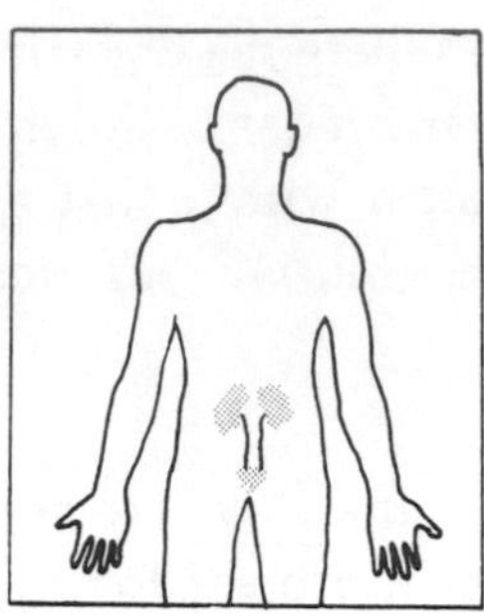

The urinary system is comprised of the kidneys, ureter tubes and the bladder. It is the chief disposal unit of the body.

KIDNEYS

The kidneys are the chief organs of the urinary system located about the midback. They perform many functions related to regulating fluid in the body and purifying the blood.

KIDNEY FUNCTIONS

chief eliminator

Filtration in the kidneys begins with the straining of fluid from the blood. This fluid is then separated into waste products to be excreted and vital substances to be reabsorbed.

other

The kidneys regulate the acid/alkaline balance of the body's fluids; they stimulate the production of red blood cells when needed; they watch over the amounts of salts and other substances in the blood.

URETER TUBES

The ureter tubes are the link between the kidneys and the bladder. They are narrow and elastic passageways through which urine passes after having been produced in the kidneys.

BLADDER

The bladder acts as a reservoir. When it is full of urine, nerve fibers react to initiate urination.

THE CIRCULATORY SYSTEM

In a general sense, the circulatory system is responsible for the constant flow of blood and other body fluids. The heart is a pump whose action keeps the blood circulating, carrying nutrients, hormones, vitamins, antibodies, heat and oxygen to the tissues and taking away all waste materials.

The circulatory system consists of the heart, blood vessels (arteries, veins, capillaries) and the lymphatic system. The lymphatic system acts as an auxiliary to the venous system.

THE HEART

The heart is the most amazing pump in the world. Every day it beats about one hundred thousand times, pumping the equivalent of eighteen hundred gallons of blood through some sixty thousand miles of blood vessels. It is a hollow, muscular organ in the chest no bigger than a clenched fist.

HEART FUNCTIONS

The sole function of the heart is to pump blood from the veins into the arteries.

LUNGS

Each lung is a network of hollow tubes and sacs which remove oxygen from the air in exchange for carbon dioxide. The lungs are located above the diaphragm in the chest. Breathing is effected when the diaphragm muscle pulls down enlarging the chest cavity and causing air to be drawn into the lungs.

THE LYMPHATIC SYSTEM

Spleen
Thymus
Lymphatic Drain

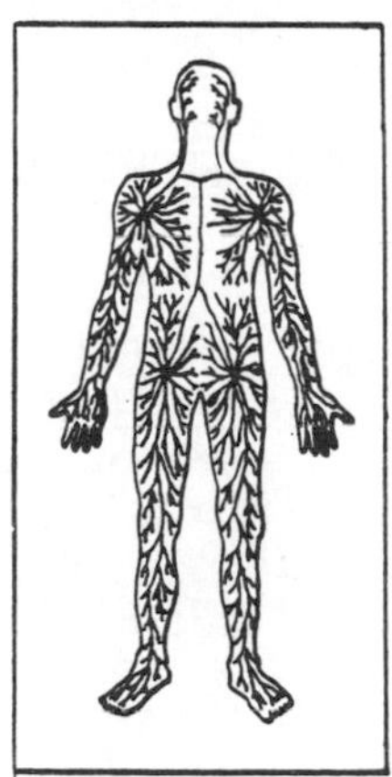

The lymphatic system is a network of thin walled vessels found in all parts of the body except the central nervous system. These vessels contain the lymph fluid which bathes all of the body's cells, feeding them with the nutrients removed by the small intestine. The fluid is filtered through little balls of cells called lymph nodes. These nodes are located mainly in the groin, armpit and neck.

LYMPHATIC FUNCTIONS

fighting infection

The lymph nodes are small "fortresses" where the lymph fluid deposits bacteria or foreign matter for disposal. In the nodes the infectious material is encapsulated and ingested by lymphocytes which produce antibodies. These antibodies are the body's chief defense against infection.

waste removal

The lymphatic system works in partnership with the venous system to effectively transport wastes produced by cell metabolism. Large particles, such as old debris of dead tissues, protein molecules and dead bacteria, cannot pass from the tissues directly into the blood through the small pores of the capillaries. The lymphatic is an accessory system taking care of those materials.

edema

The lymph fluid is not pumped throughout the body by any heartlike organ, but is pressed forward by contractions of surrounding muscles. Lymph fluid can pool in the legs and feet, which then swell. This pooling can be caused by a plugged lymph node, heart disorders, too much salt in the diet or as a side effect of medication.

SPLEEN

The spleen is an organ in the abdomen cupping the left edge of the pancreas and is part of the lymphatic system.

SPLEEN FUNCTIONS

manufacturing lymphocytes

The spleen produces antibodies and filters the lymph fluids in the same way as a lymph node.

blood cell quality control

The spleen removes and destroys faulty or deformed red blood cells and recycles iron for hemoglobin production. Hemoglobin is the substance which carries oxygen to the tissues. The spleen also is a reservoir for the storage of extra blood.

DYSFUNCTIONS CONTROLLED BY THE SPLEEN

The spleen is involved in various widespread disorders of the lymphoid and blood forming tissues, e.g. leukemia, Hodgkin's disease and anemia.

THYMUS

The thymus is a lymph gland located behind the upper part of the breastbone.

FUNCTIONS

The thymus plays a key role in the development of the immune system in infants. It appears to continue to play an important part in the body's immune system throughout life.

maturation and development of the immune system

THE LYMPHATIC DRAIN

The lymphatic system finally drains its fluid into two veins at the base of the neck.

The waste and excess fluid is removed from the blood by the kidneys and eliminated by urination. These veins are important for the transition of the lymph fluid into the venous system.

THE CENTRAL NERVOUS SYSTEM

The nervous system, in general, regulates rapid muscular and secretory activities of the body, whereas the hormonal system (endocrine) regulates mainly the slowly reacting metabolic functions. The central nervous system consists of the brain, spinal cord and the nerves emanating from them.

THE BRAIN AND THE CRANIAL NERVES

The brain consists of two hemispheres. The left controls the right half of the body and vice versa. This "crossover" is important to reflexologists in that it is the major exception to zone theory. In zone theory the right foot represents the right half of the body, and the left foot the left half. Disorders involving one side of the brain will appear as dysfunction on the opposite side of the body. In the case of a stroke, for example, the large toe on the opposite side from the paralysis will be more sensitive.

The brain is the central computer that controls both the voluntary and involuntary system of the body. In other words it controls the central nervous system and the endocrine system, both of which jointly control the complex activities of the whole body.

There are twelve pairs of cranial nerves arising from the brain and passing through the holes in the skull. Some of the cranial nerves are only sensory (taste, smell, sight and hearing), but the majority are motor nerves. Probably the most important of the cranial nerves is the vagus nerve. It is the largest nerve in the body supplying the heart, lungs and abdominal organs.

SPINAL CORD AND SPINAL NERVES

The spinal cord is the continuation of the brain below the skull. It is a column of nervous tissue enclosed in the spinal canal, a tunnel in the backbone. The nerves originating from the spinal cord are channels for conveying information from the peripheral nerves of the body and to the muscles and glands.

The cervical nerves control the neck and arms. The thoracic portion provides nerves to the chest. The lumbar nerves are distributed to the lower extremities, the legs and feet, and the sacral nerves mainly supply the organs of the pelvis, the pelvic and buttock muscles.

The spinal nerves are named and numbered according to the vertebral divisions of the spinal column into cervical, thoracic, lumbar and sacral segments.

The spine has seven cervicals starting with the atlas-axis (the first and second cervicals which is what the head pivots on). It ends with the seventh cervical, a protruding vertebrae at the base of the neck.

The seventh cervical effects everything down into the fingertips (see numbness pg. 134).

From the seventh cervical down are the twelve thoracic vertebrae each carrying a pair of ribs. These end at the waistline which marks the beginning of the five lumbar vertebrae. This is the lower back. The lower back has a profound effect on everything in that region such as the reproductive organs, digestive tract and the lower limbs.

Below the lumbar vertebrae are five fused vertebrae which form the sacrum and the vestiges of the tail, the coccyx. This area can affect many parts including the head (when headaches occur).

THE HEAD

The head accommodates the brain, several sense organs, and inlets for air and food. Disorders of the brain, eyes, ears, and sinus cavities are of greatest interest to reflexologists because they are the most commonly encountered.

THE EARS

The ears gather the vibrations from the air and turn them into meaningful messages.

The outer shell of the ear only captures the sound. The actual mechanism for hearing is well protected in the head.

The sound travels down a tunnel into the middle ear, which is enclosed in a membrane called the eardrum. The eardrum flutters in response to sound.

A fine set of bones called the hammer, anvil and stirrup are attached to the inside of the eardrum. The eardrum vibrations make these bones move in response, transmitting their message to the inner ear.

The inner ear houses apparatuses for two separate functions. The cochlea takes the vibrations and translates them into nerve messages. The semicircular canals housed with the cochlea are responsible for our balance.

THE EYES

The eyes act like a camera taking in the view and sending the message to the brain.

A lens focuses light into the eye. The light travels to the back of the eye shining on a fine nerve network of cells called the retina. The retina triggers a signal of what it sees to the optic nerve. The message is relayed through the second cranial nerve to the brain where it is interpreted.

MUSCULAR SYSTEM

Muscle is the most abundant tissue in the body. It accounts for some two fifths of the body weight. There are two involuntary types of muscles: the smooth muscles (found in the walls of digestive and urinary tract, other hollow organs, and the blood vessels) and the cardiac muscles (muscles of the heart). The striated muscles are voluntary muscles but they also take part in unconscious reflexes.

Muscles have essentially two actions: contraction and relaxation. The range of these two actions are important for the body's return to equilibrium. Chemicals essential to contracting the muscles to meet certain challenges can be left over, causing residual tension. Residual tension in these muscles can have effects on the skeletal system, organs, glands, and circulatory systems.

SKELETAL SYSTEM

The bones of the body are not a static structure. They store nearly all of the body's reserves of calcium. They also manufacture red blood cells (a function performed by red bone marrow).

The skeleton provides a firm framework giving shape to the body and its parts. It supports and protects vital parts such as the heart, brain and lungs from injury. The skeleton facilitates body movements by acting in cooperation with various muscles attached to the bones by tendons.

TABLE OF DISORDERS
(Suggested Areas of Emphasis)

The following table is a guide to suggested areas of emphasis for various disorders. The areas are listed in descending order of importance. It should only serve as a guide and is not a diagnostic tool. The whole foot should be worked if possible.

DISORDER	QUICK REFERENCE	
Allergies	Adrenal glands (pp.40-42) Reproductive glands (pp.52-53) Pituitary (p. 30)	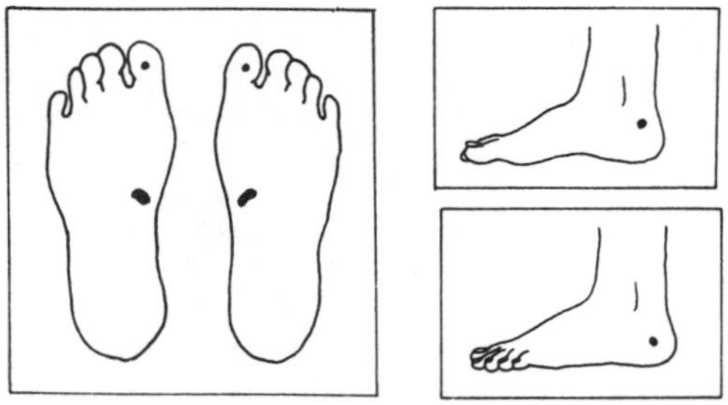
Anemia	Spleen (pp.40-42)	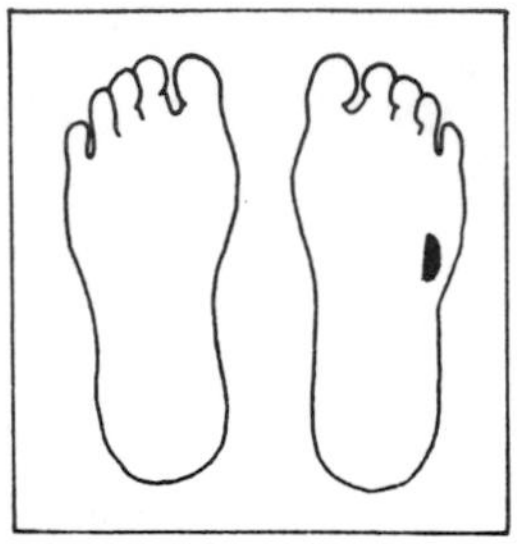
Angina-Pectoris	Heart (pp.37-39) Adrenal Glands (pp.40-42) Chest Area (pp.37-39)	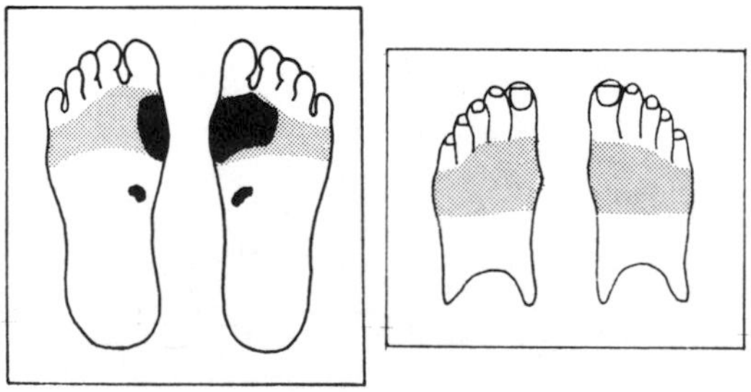

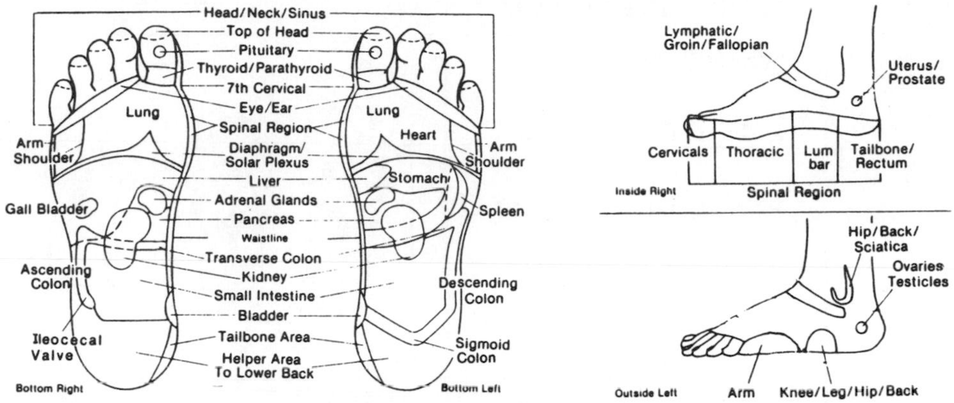

DESCRIPTION AND EMPHASIS

A misuse of immunity, a defense against infection in times of no danger. It is overreaction by the body's defense mechanisms to certain food, clothing, pollen and other materials.

The adrenal glands are important in anything involving an inflammation created when the body's defenses misconstrue certain materials. Because they also have endocrine functions aside from their reproductive functions, the reproductive glands are helpful. The pituitary governs the other endocrine glands with its hormones.

A lack of iron in the blood cells. The spleen, as a recycler of iron, is important in the manufacture of hemoglobin. Hemoglobin is an iron-containing protein in the red blood cells, responsible for carrying oxygen from the lungs to the body tissues.

A pain in the chest caused by a spasm of the coronary arteries of the heart.

Work the heart area thoroughly on both top and bottom of both feet. Pay particular attention to the troughs between the first and second toes.

DISORDER	QUICK REFERENCE	
Arthritis	Whole Foot Kidneys (pp.40-42,44) Adrenal Glands (pp.40-42) Solar Plexus (p. 36)	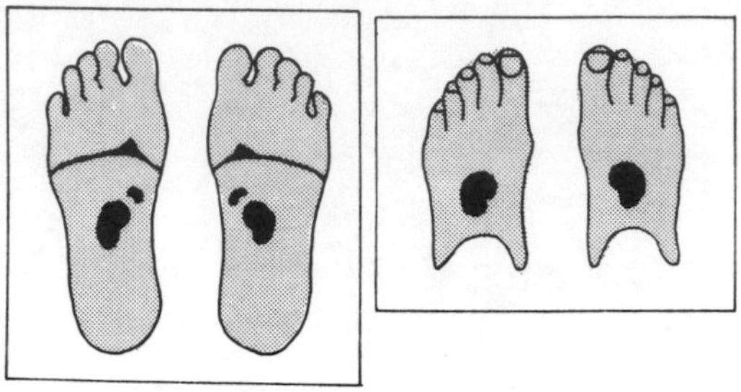
Asthma	Adrenal Glands (pp.40-42) Ileocecal Valve (pp.44-45) Solar Plexus (p. 36) Lungs (pp.37-39)	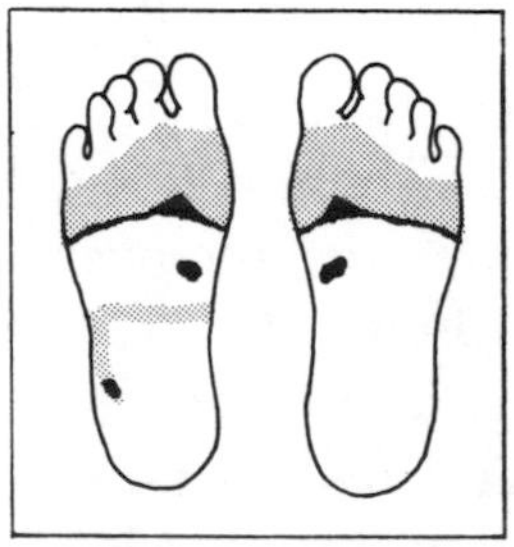
Atrophy of the Optic Nerve	Eyes (pp.35-36) Kidneys (pp.40-42,44) Neck (pp.32-34)	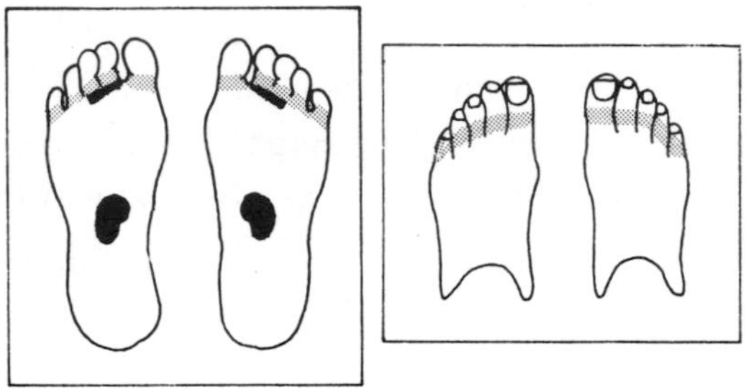
Back Disorders	Spine (pp.47-48)	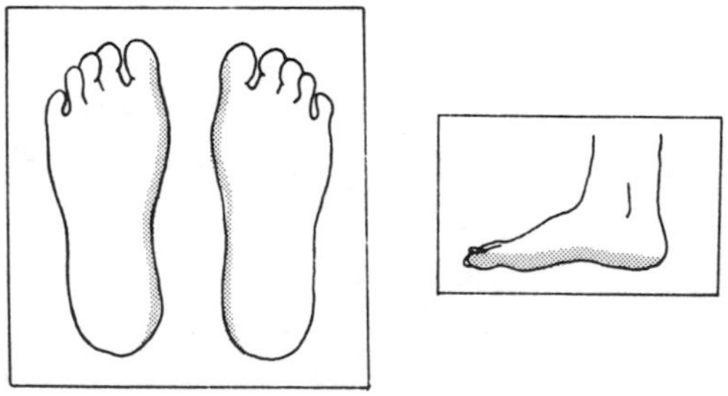

DESCRIPTION AND EMPHASIS
A general body condition coming from a variety of sources and generally associated with an inflammation of a joint. Because it is a general body condition, the whole foot should be worked. The kidneys can be useful in eliminating waste materials which can gather around the joints. The adrenal glands' inflammation fighting qualities are important. According to recent studies, tension has an effect on arthritis. Working the solar plexus area for relaxation of tension may help the root cause of arthritis.
An allergic condition associated with wheezing, coughing, and difficulty in exhaling. Adrenalin is administered by a doctor for asthma attacks. The adrenal glands produce their own adrenalin and this area on the feet is emphasized for asthma. The ileocecal valve area is worked for the control of mucus. Working the solar plexus area eases the tension that often accompanies an attack.
A degeneration of the nerve fibers for a variety of reasons. A loss of vision results.
Support structure for the body and housing structure for the spinal cord, the continuation of the brain below the skull. The spine (and its influence) go beyond its role as a supporting structure. The nerves originating from the spinal cord assert control over large segments of the torso. (See Sciatica)

DISORDER	QUICK REFERENCE	
Neck (Cervicals)	Neck (pp.32-34) Tops of Shoulders (p. 34) Solar Plexus (p. 36)	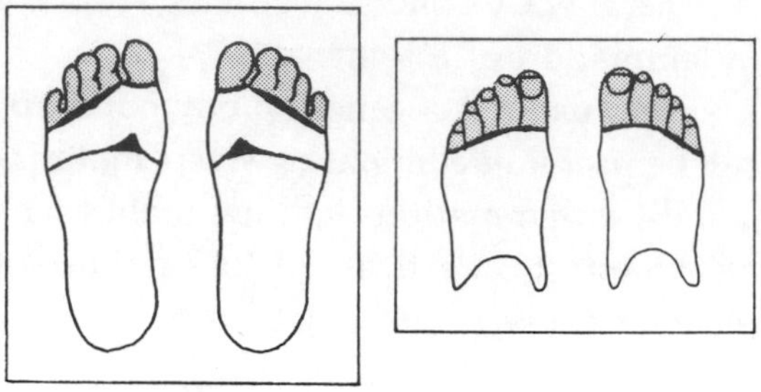
Mid Back (Thoracics)	Spine (pp.47-48) Solar Plexus (p. 36)	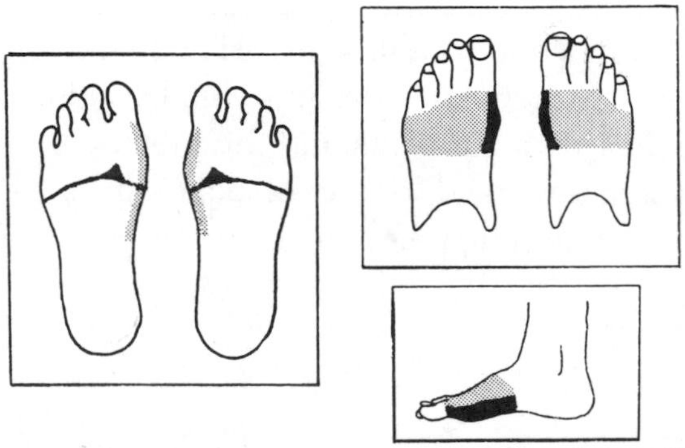
Lower back (Lumbars)	Spine (pp.47-48) Hip (p. 49) Solar Plexus (p. 36) Knee/Leg (p. 50) Lymph/Groin (p. 51)	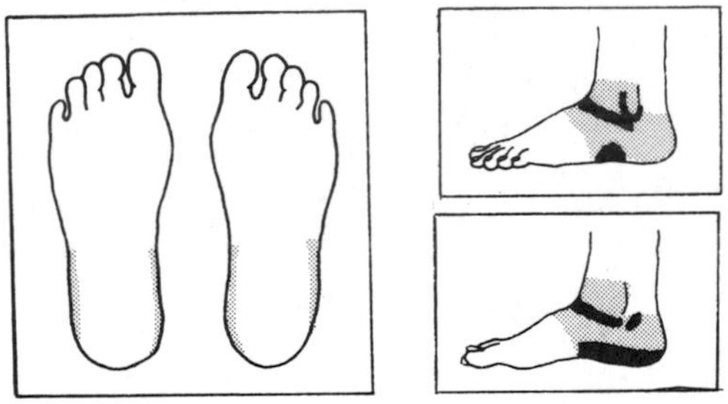
Lower Back (Tailbone)	Spine (pp.47-48) Lumbars (pp.48-50)	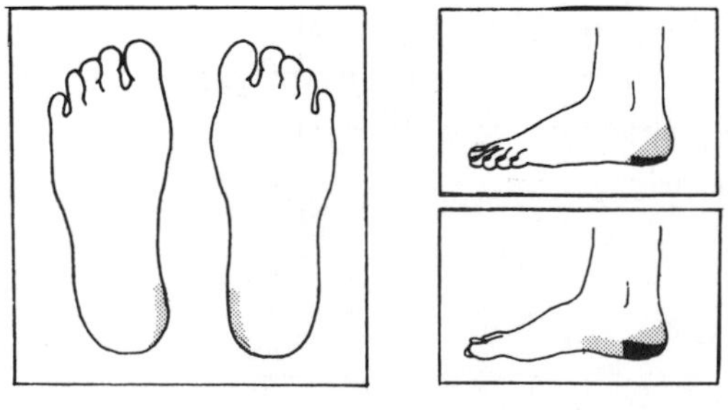
Back *See also*	*Hip Disorders* *Sciatica*	

DESCRIPTION AND EMPHASIS
The seven cervicals of the neck are likely to be affected by tension and injuries and their resulting problems are common. For cervical problems work all sides of every toe, paying particular attention to the big toe. The cervicals are located on several lateral zones, with the seventh cervical encompassing the circular band at the base of the toe. The shoulders and solar plexus should be worked in the appropriate areas on the feet because they, too, are areas commonly concerned with tension.
The vertebrae attached to the ribs are involved in upper back problems from the neck to the waistline. The spinal area from the base of the big toe to the "waistline" on the foot should be worked. This area wraps around the inside of the foot. An accompanying area is the solar plexus (tension).
These five lumbar vertebrae bear much of the body's weight and therefore are subject to many problems. Work the area from the waistline into the hollow of the heel. Puffiness in the hollow can be indicative of lower back or bladder problems, two overlapping areas. The lower back is interrelated with and can cause problems in many other areas. They should all be worked in conjunction with a problem in any one.
The area on the foot runs from the hollow of the heel down the inside edge of the heel. Helper areas include: areas on both inside and outside of the heel extending into the ankle, the heel area on the bottom of the foot, and the lumbars.

DISORDER	QUICK REFERENCE	
Bladder Disorders	Bladder (pp.47-48) Kidney (pp.40-42,44) Ureter Tubes (pp.40-42,44)	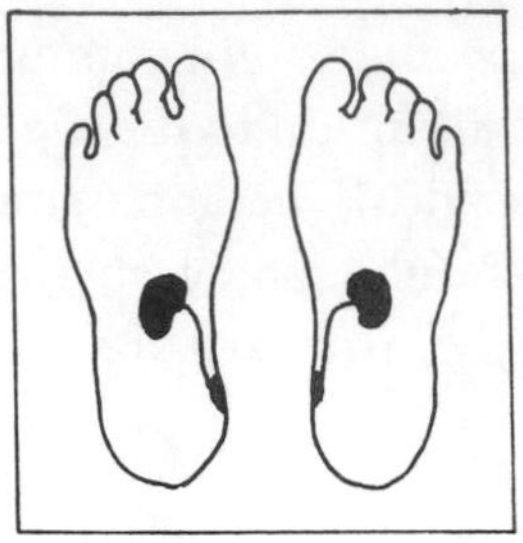
Breast	Chest (pp.37-39) Lymphatic Glands (p. 51) Pituitary (p. 30)	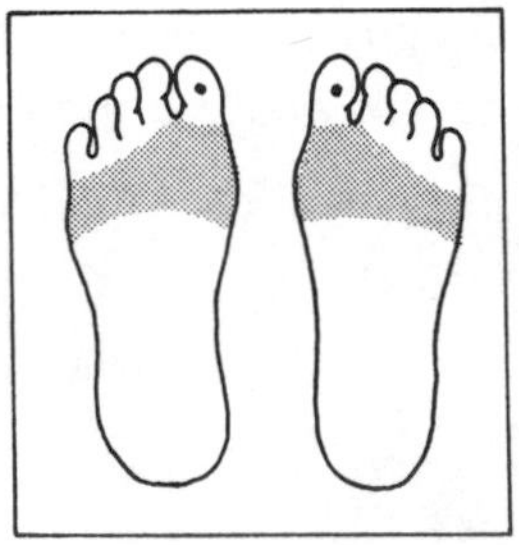 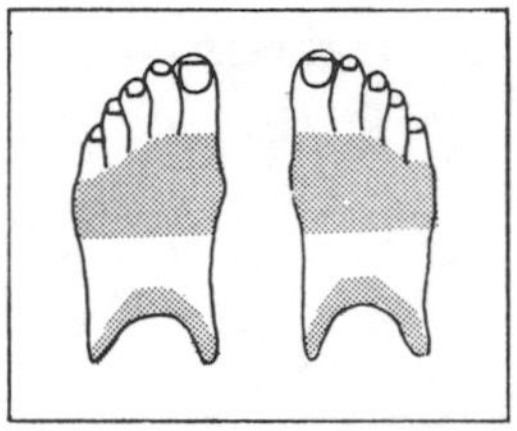
Bursitis	Shoulder (if affected) (pp.37-39) Adrenal Glands (pp.40-42)	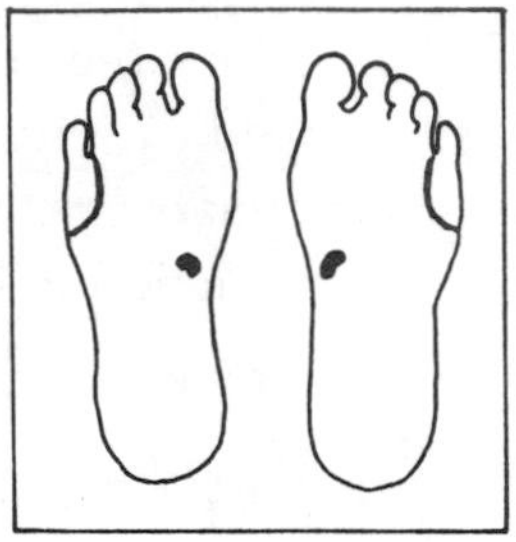
Callouses **Callouses** *See Also*	*Corns*	

DESCRIPTION AND EMPHASIS
Reservoir for holding urine. The bladder/lower back areas overlap and are located in the hollow of the heel (See Lower Back). Puffiness here may indicate problems in the bladder or lower back. Check the whole urinary system area (kidneys, ureter tubes) as well.
The breasts can be considered part of the lymphatic system as lymph nodes are spread throughout the breast area. The lymphatic nodes drain the fat portion of the milk during lactation. They are a vehicle for transferring infection to more distant parts. Plugged lymph nodes rather than malignancies are responsible for the majority of lumps detected. The pituitary area is worked for any type of growth.
Bursitis is an inflammation of the bursa, a soft tissue sac that lies between body parts that move on each other (especially in joints). The shoulders are often susceptible to this problem. Working the adrenal glands areas on both feet can be helpful with the inflammation. If the inflammation exists in other areas, work the referral areas (See pg. 12) on the body.
A thickening in the outermost layer of skin in response to friction or pressure. Hard callouses may not have much sensitivity at the surface but below these heavy pads lie important reflexes. Frequently these reflexes are heavily built up with deposits as they are insulated from external stimulus. Work right through the callouses. Thick callouses may require the attention of a podiatrist. As with corns, sensitive callouses should be worked carefully. Working the area around a callous stimulates circulation in that area. Work cautiously through the callous itself.

DISORDER	QUICK REFERENCE	
Cataracts	Eye/Ear (pp.35-36) Kidneys (pp.40-42,44) Neck (pp.32-34)	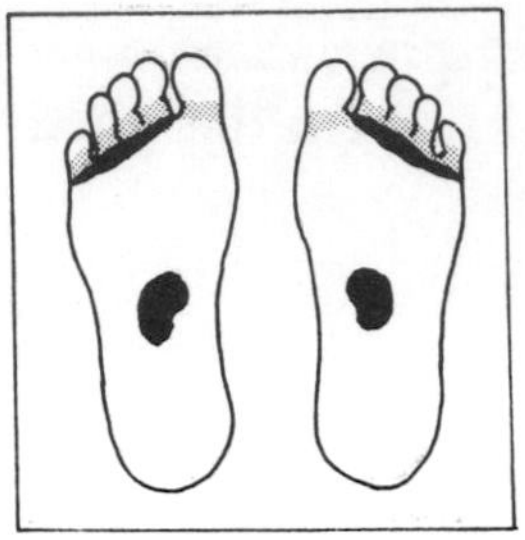
Colitis	Colon (pp.44-46) Solar Plexus (p. 36) Adrenal Glands (pp.40-42)	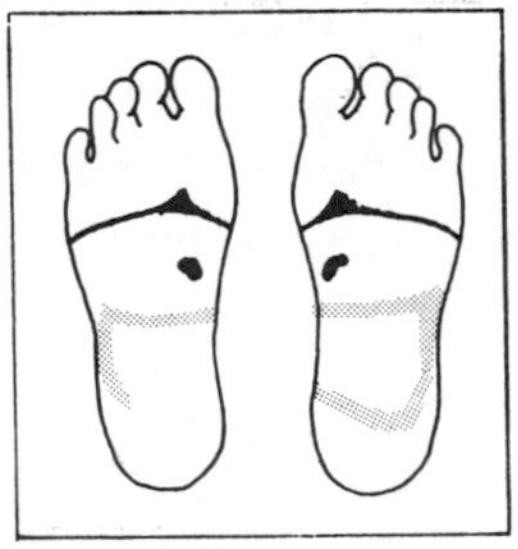
Constipation	Colon (pp.44-46) Liver/Gall Bladder (pp.40-42) Adrenal Glands (pp.40-42) Solar Plexus (p. 36) Lower Back (pp.48-50)	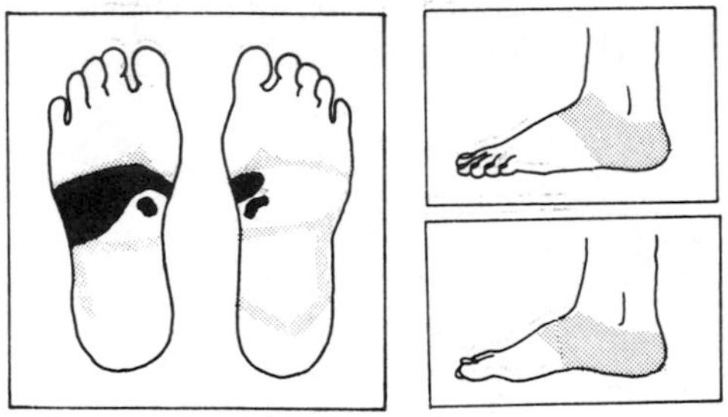
Corns		

DESCRIPTION AND EMPHASIS
Cataracts are growths over the lens of the eye; the lens becomes opaque. They generally occur in old age but can also occur as a result of injury. In rare cases cataracts may be present at birth. The earlier they are detected, the better the chances for successful treatment. The eye/ear reflex areas need thorough attention. When the lens becomes totally grown over and surgery becomes necessary, it is still important to work the eye/ear area and other associated areas. This assists the healing process and helps control the scarring that accompanies surgery. Since these areas lie in the same zones as the kidney areas, use each as a referral area to help the other. Tension in the neck can also cause eye/ear problems. Work neck areas thoroughly.
An inflammation of the colon. It is important to find on the foot the area that relates to the irritation in the colon. Tension is often involved in digestive problems. Work the solar plexus area for tension and the adrenals for inflammation.
Constipation arises from a variety of sources including tension. The liver and gall bladder produce and store the bile needed for digestion. The adrenal glands are essential to smooth muscle operation (as in the peristaltic ((muscle)) contraction of the digestive system). Problems in the lower back can affect everything within its area. The digestive system is also vulnerable to the side effects of tension. The areas on the feet corresponding to these parts of the body should be worked.
Corns are formed in response to increased pressure or friction, causing irritation to the nerve endings. Working with corns requires common sense and caution. Work around the fringes of the corn to bring back circulation. Make several light passes through the area. Corns can be extremely sensitive and should be worked to the person's level of tolerance.

DISORDER	QUICK REFERENCE	
Depression	Endocrine Glands (pp.40-42, 52-53) Solar Plexus (p. 36) Pancreas (pp.40-42) Head (pp.32-34)	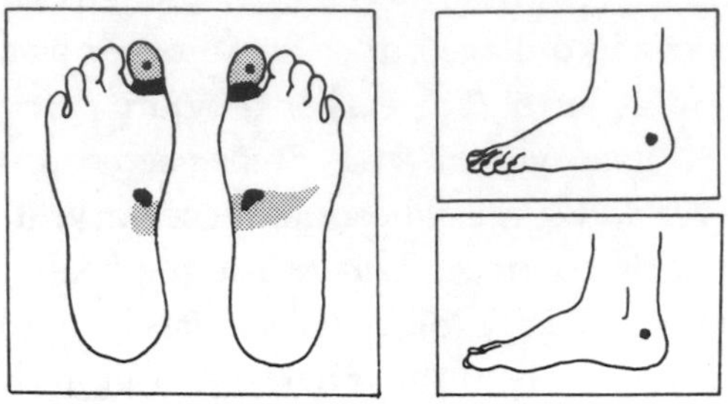
Detached Retina	Eye/Ear (pp.35-36) Neck (pp.32-34) Kidneys (pp.40-42,44)	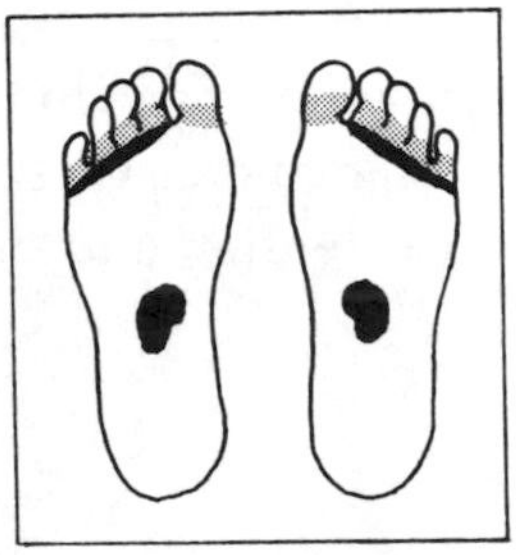
Diabetes	Pancreas (pp.40-42) Pituitary (p. 30) Thyroid (p. 31) Liver (pp.40-42) Adrenal Glands (pp.40-42)	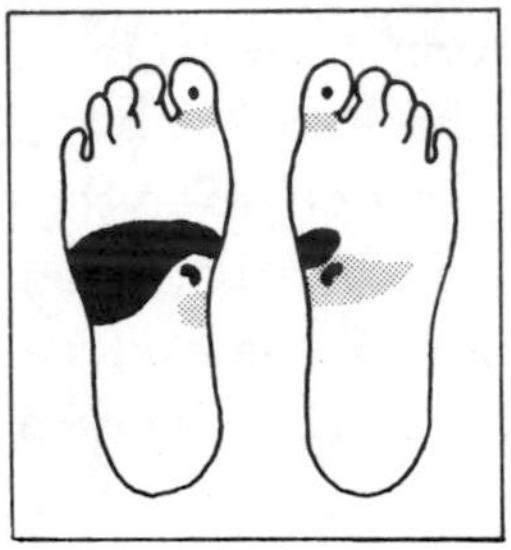
Diabetes *See Also*	*Hypoglycemia*	
Digestive Disorders	*See* *Colitis* *Constipation* *Diverticulitis* *Flatulence* *Hemorrhoids* *Hiatal Hernia* *Ulcers*	

DESCRIPTION AND EMPHASIS
The factors contributing to depression can be psychological or physical. Among physical factors are the endocrine glands and their effects on the vigor and degree of activity. Another factor can be tension as a potential source of depression or as a complicating element. Blood sugar levels have been suspected in mood fluctuations. The pancreas is involved in controlling the blood sugar level with insulin.
Separation of the retina from the outer layers of the eyeball resulting in partial or total blindness. If surgery is necessary, work the areas listed above before and after to help the healing process.
This is a disease characterized by the body's inability to burn up sugars (carbohydrates) that have been consumed. An insufficient production of insulin is responsible. Insulin is a hormone produced by cells in the pancreas, which secretes it into the blood, permitting the metabolism and utilization of sugar. If this secretion is insufficient, the blood sugar level rises rapidly causing a series of dangerous conditions. The reverse of this condition is hypoglycemia (See pg. 96). Frequent urination (an attempt to rid the blood of excess glucose), loss of weight (an attempt to burn fat instead of glucose) and degeneration of small vessels (particularly in the eyes and kidneys) are symptomatic of diabetes. It can lead to blindness and kidney disease. Circulatory problems frequently complicate this condition. Juvenile diabetes is the severe form of this disease. The pituitary as the master endocrine gland effects the pancreas. The thyroid, liver, and adrenal glands play a role in metabolism. Work these areas thoroughly.

DISORDER	QUICK REFERENCE	
Diverticulitis	Colon (pp.44-46) Sigmoid Colon (p. 46) Solar Plexus (p. 36) Adrenal Glands (pp.40-42)	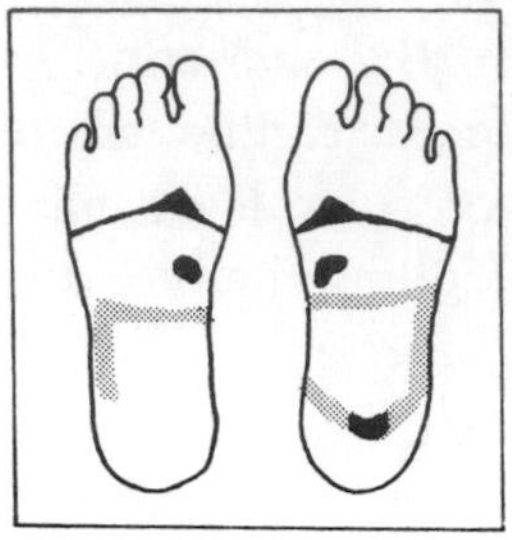
Dizziness (Vertigo)	Eye/Ear (pp.35-36)	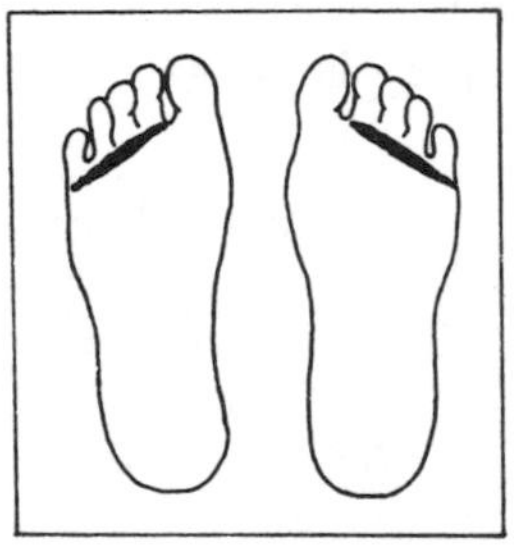
Earache	Eye/Ear (pp.35-36)	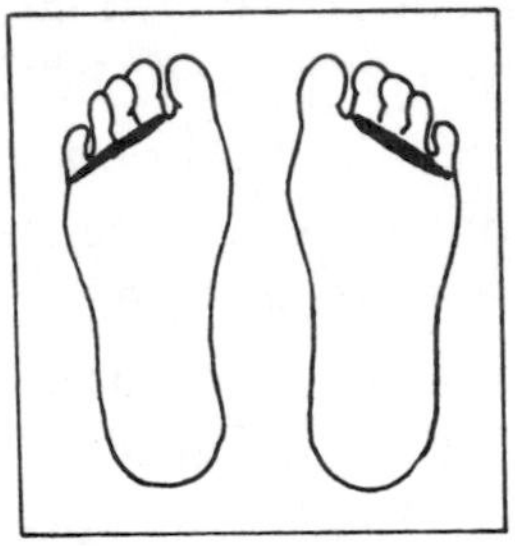
Eczema	Endocrine Glands (pp.40-42, 52-53) Solar Plexus (p. 36) Kidneys (pp.40-42,44) Lymph (p. 51)	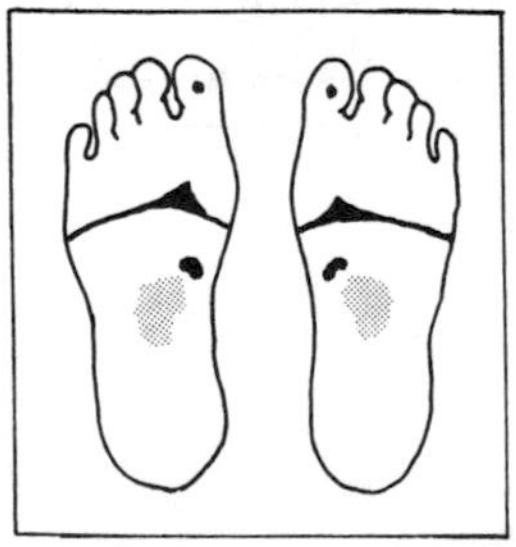 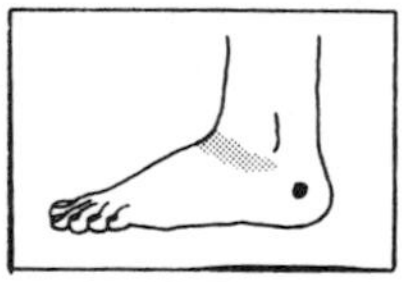 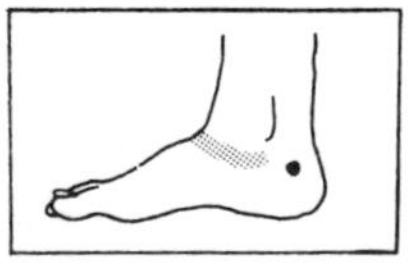

DESCRIPTION AND EMPHASIS
The diverticulum is a sac arising from the bowel wall. Diverticulitis is the condition in which this sac becomes inflamed. This disorder is fairly common around the lower colon area. Work the entire colon areas on the feet, paying particular attention to the sigmoid colon. Work the adrenal glands for inflammation.
The causes of dizziness are varied. A common cause is an infection of the inner ear which contains the mechanism for balance. Vertigo describes a condition in which the room seems to be spinning. For these problems carefully probe the eye/ear areas on the feet, checking the neck areas for any tenderness.
Earache — Infection is a prime cause of earache. Check the toes for soreness in the neck areas. Work the eye/ear areas thoroughly, giving added emphasis to the adrenal glands when inflammation or infection is involved.
Eczema is a disorder involving dryness of skin. The thyroid and adrenal glands areas have often been found to be helpful with this disorder. The skin contributes to the waste elimination process. Working the lymphatic and kidney areas helps the problem by easing some of this burden.

DISORDER	QUICK REFERENCE	
Emphysema	Lung (pp.37-39) Ileocecal (pp.44-45) Solar Plexus (p. 36)	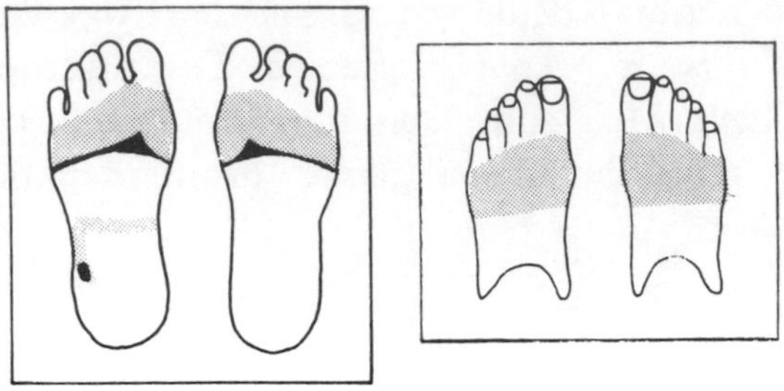
Eye Disorders	Eye/Ear (pp.35-36) Neck (pp.32-34) Kidneys (pp.40-42,44)	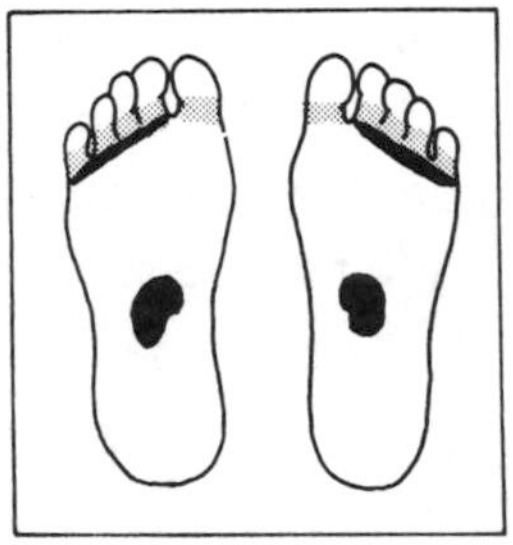
Eye Disorders *See Also*	*Atrophy of the Optic Nerve* *Cataracts* *Detached Retina* *Glaucoma*	
Fainting	Pituitary (p. 30)	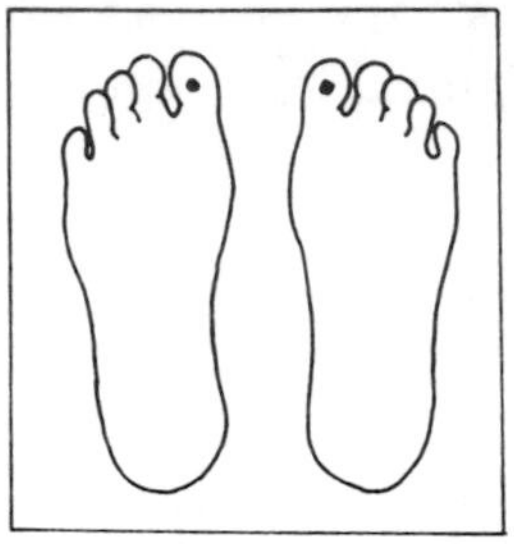
Female Disorders	Uterus (pp.52-53) Ovary (pp.52-53) Fallopian Tubes (p. 51)	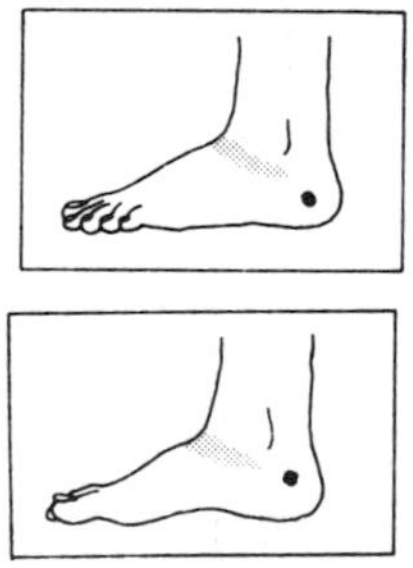
Female Disorders *See Also*	*Hysterectomy* *Infertility*	

DESCRIPTION AND EMPHASIS
Emphysema is a lung condition in which exhaling is difficult. The lung sac becomes inelastic. Tension is also a major contributor to this problem. Excess mucus aggravates the situation even further. Cover the lung areas on the feet thoroughly. Also emphasize the ileocecal valve area for mucus and the solar plexus area for tension.
Work the eye/ear areas at the base of the toes for all eye disorders. The neck is a good helper area to eye problems because the blood and nerve supply passes through it. Because of the zonal relationship (See pg. 11) the kidney areas provide additional aid.
Fainting is caused by sudden insufficient blood supply to the brain. It is sometimes possible to revive an unconscious person who has just fainted by working the pituitary area of both big toes using the *thumb hook and back up* technique (See page 29) repeatedly. After the person is revived, work the rest of the foot to help eliminate the cause of the fainting.
The female reproductive areas include the uterus, the ovaries and the fallopian tubes which join them. These areas are commonly affected by menstrual problems, menopause, and infertility. Areas to emphasize on the feet include all of the reproductive areas and the endocrine glands because of the interrelationship of all the glands. For menstrual problems and menopause the above areas are important with special emphasis on the uterus area. Infertility can be caused by infection, blocked fallopian tube, endocrine gland dysfunction, or psychological problems. Thus all of the reproductive areas and the other endocrine gland areas are important ones to emphasize. A hysterectomy is a surgical removel of the uterus. The uterus area still needs attention because of the ensuing scar tissue and adhesions.

DISORDER	QUICK REFERENCE	
Fever	Pituitary (p. 30)	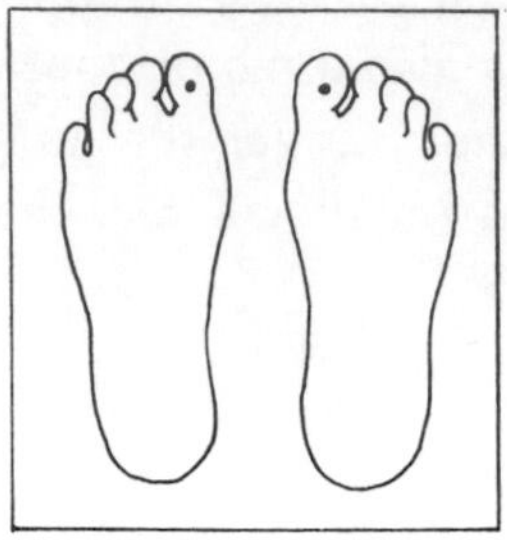
Flatulence	Sigmoid Colon (p. 46) Solar Plexus (p. 36) Intestine (p. 45)	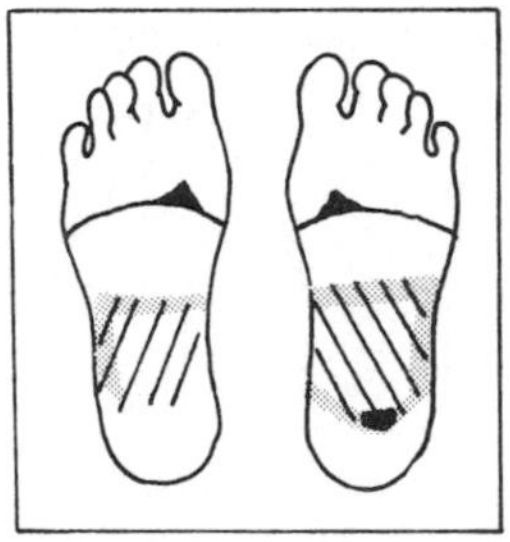
Gallstones	Liver/Gallbladder (pp.40-42)	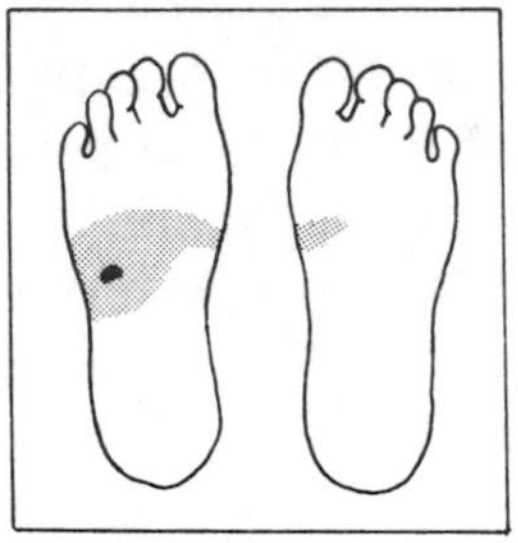
Glaucoma	Eye/Ear (pp.35-36) Neck (pp.32-34) Kidney (pp.40-42,44)	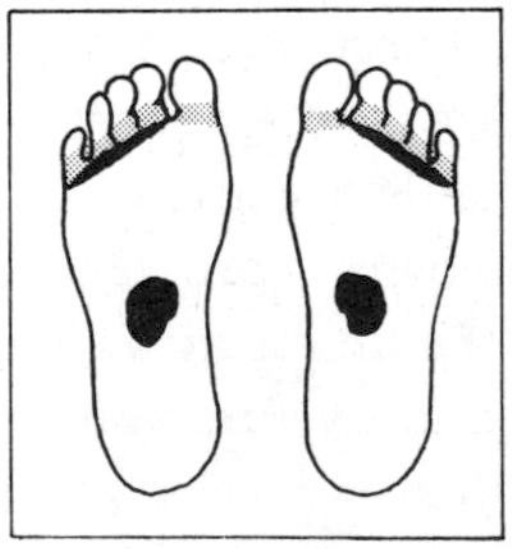

Glaucoma *See Also* *Eye Disorders*

DESCRIPTION AND EMPHASIS
Increase in body temperature associated with infection (also a symptom of other illnesses). Work only the pituitary area every half an hour until the fever is reduced, then work the rest of the foot.
An excessive accumulation of gas in the stomach or intestine. The sigmoid colon, because of its location, is a prime target for flatulence. On the feet the sigmoid colon, the intestines and solar plexus areas should be worked.
Crystallized fatty particles particularly cholesterol. The size of a gallstone can be as small as a seed to as large as a lemon. The larger the gallstone the greater the potential for problems. Work the liver/gallbladder areas thoroughly.
An eye disease associated with increased pressure of the fluid in the eyeball, leading to blindness if left untreated. It is usually not painful. Routine glaucoma examinations are now commonplace and therefore the disease can be detected and treated early. As in most disorders, long-term glaucoma will require more time to get results with reflexology. The eye/ear area should be probed thoroughly. As with all eye problems, the neck and kidney areas on the feet should be emphasized. High blood pressure or hypertension (See pg. 130) is a side effect of the eye drops used to treat glaucoma.

DISORDER	QUICK REFERENCE	
Gout	Kidneys (pp.40-42,44) Corresponding body area	
Gout *See Also*	*Kidney Disorders*	
Hard of Hearing *See* *Hearing Disorders*		
Hardening of the Arteries *See* *Hypertension*		
Hay Fever	Adrenal Glands (pp.40-42) Reproductive Glands (pp.52-53) Pituitary (p. 30) Head/Neck/Sinus (pp.32-34) Ileocecal Valve (pp.44-45)	
Hay Fever *See Also*	*Allergies*	
Headaches	Head/neck/sinus (pp.32-34) Solar Plexus (p. 36) Tailbone and Spine (pp.47-48)	
Hearing Disorders	Eye/Ear (pp.35-36) Neck (pp.32-34)	
Hearing Disorders	*See Also* *Dizziness* *Earache*	

DESCRIPTION AND EMPHASIS
Gout: An excess of uric acid in the blood which causes inflammation around a joint. Attacks are sudden and painful. The big toe is a frequent target for gout but not the only area where it can occur. The kidneys control uric acid and their areas on the feet are therefore important. Work the corresponding joint (referral area) in the hand as well.
An allergic response of the upper respiratory tract, usually to pollen in the environment. Work head/neck/sinus and ileocecal valve (for mucus) for additional help with this problem.
Headaches occur in response to certain drugs, physical conditions and even anxiety. The toes represent the head and neck area. The big toe in itself is a study for tension in the head and neck. Try working all through the head and neck areas on the feet. The solar plexus needs attention for reducing tension. Migraine is a common and particularly distressing type of headache. Migraines are not yet fully understood. The areas mentioned above are important. The spine also needs careful attention along its entire length, particularly the tailbone area. Unusual as this sounds, many migraines have been linked to injuries in this area.
Partial or complete loss of hearing due to age, accident, genetic defect, occupational hazard or other cause. The bones of the middle ear are vital and if damaged, little can be done to improve the hearing. Balance is still an important function of the ear, even when hearing is impaired or lost. As with any hearing problem, the eye/ear and neck areas should be worked.

DISORDER	QUICK REFERENCE	
Heart Attacks	Heart/Lung (pp.32-34) Adrenal Glands (pp.40-42) Sigmoid Colon (p. 46)	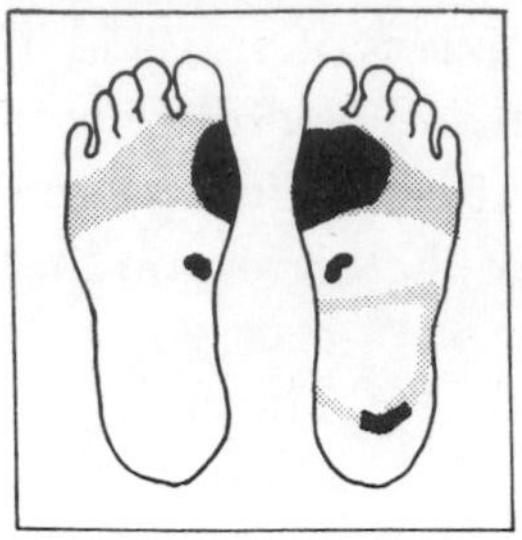
Heart Attack *See Also Hypertension*		
Heart Disorders *See Angina Pectoris*		
Hemorrhoids	Hip Region (p. 49) Lower Back (pp.48-50) Sigmoid Colon (p. 46) Solar Plexus (p. 36)	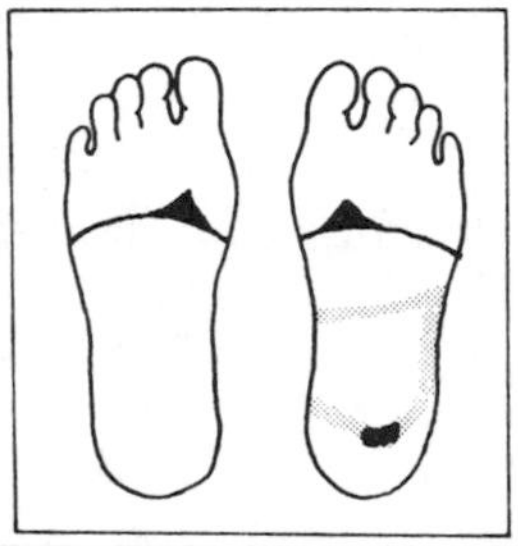 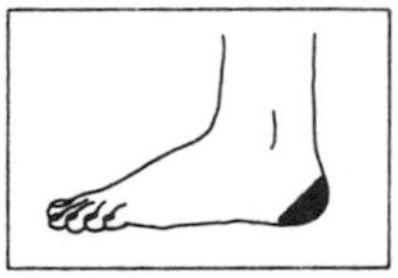 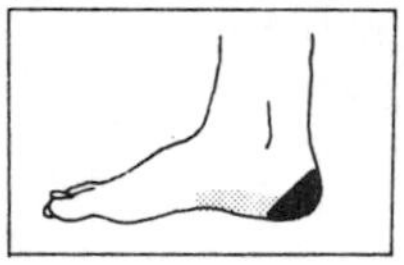
Hiatal Hernia	Solar Plexus (p. 36) Adrenal Glands (pp.40-42)	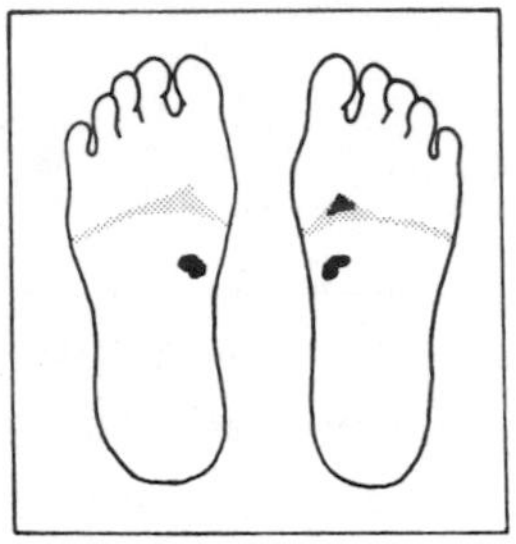
High Blood Pressure *See Hypertension* *See Also Heart Attack*		
Hip Disorders	Lymph/Groin (p. 51) Hip Region (p. 49) Hip/Back/Sciatic (p. 49) Knee/Leg (p. 50) Lower Back (pp.48-50)	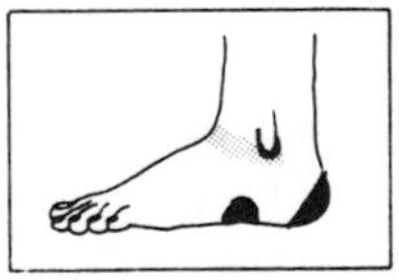 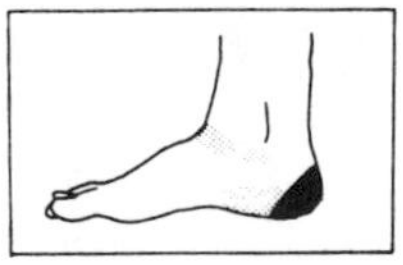
Hip Disorders *See Also Back*		

DESCRIPTION AND EMPHASIS
An obstruction of the coronary artery or one of its branches by a blood clot, depriving part of the heart muscle of blood. The heart area extends across the ball of the left foot and onto part of the right foot as well. The entire heart/lung area needs emphasis. The heart is a muscle and the adrenal glands can help with muscle tone. The sigmoid colon is one part of the intestine particularly prone to the trapping and pocketing of gas. This increased pressure can back up along the colon to the transverse section where it can put pressure on the chest cavity.
Hemorrhoids are varicose veins of the rectum. At times the colon itself actually becomes extended outward. Work the lower back/tailbone area. This includes all the areas around the heel (particularly where the shoe meets the back of the foot). The bottom of the heels, particularly the sigmoid colon area, can be of value. Tension may be part of the problem. Work the solar plexus areas.
A hernia of the diaphragm taking place at the opening through which the esophagus passes. It is a ballooning of the diaphragm wall. The diaphragm is a strong layer of muscle and fibrous tissue dividing the chest and the abdominal cavities. People often complain of indigestion because a spasm in the sphincter valve leading to the stomach allows acid to splash up into the unprotected esophagus. The esophagus runs to the left as it enters the stomach, so the left foot will tend to be more sensitive than the right in the solar plexus area. Sharp pain will often be encountered here. Work the diaphragm/solar plexus area completely, emphasizing the adrenal glands for muscle tone.
Hip problems have a variety of sources. The lower back is frequently the root cause of this problem. Search the hip region, the hip/back/sciatic, lymph/groin and knee/leg for sensitive areas.

DISORDER	QUICK REFERENCE	
Hypertension	Solar Plexus (p. 36) Adrenal Glands (pp.40-42) Kidneys (pp.40-42,44)	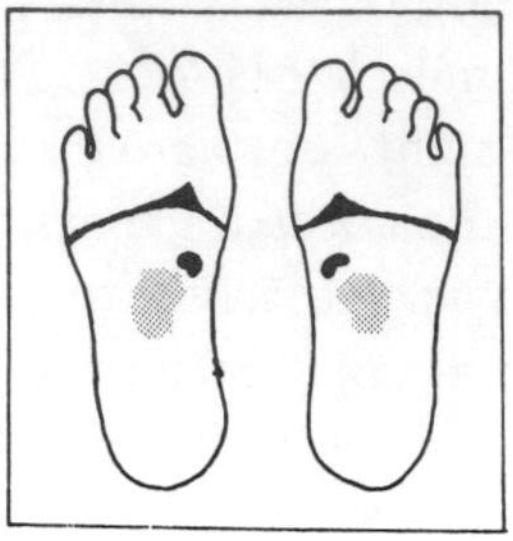
Hypertension *See Also*	*Colitis* *Ulcers*	
Hypoglycemia	Pancreas (pp.40-42) Pituitary (p. 30) Thyroid (p. 31) Liver (pp.40-42) Adrenal Glands (pp.40-42)	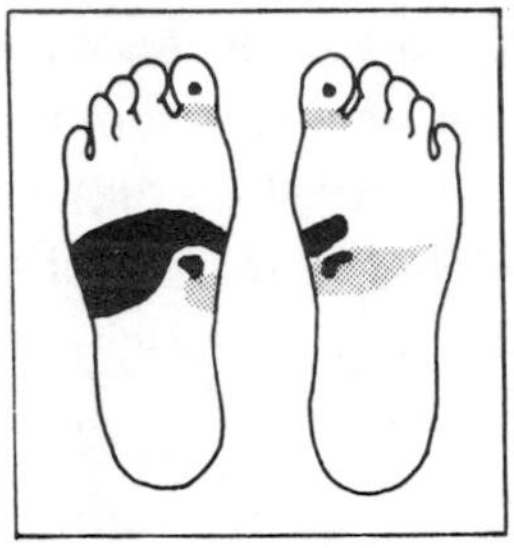
Hypoglycemia *See Also*	*Depression* *Diabetes*	
Hysterectomy *See*	*Female Disorders*	

DESCRIPTION AND EMPHASIS
A condition in which the heart is forced to pump under higher pressure which puts excessive strain on it. It can speed up the development of atherosclerosis (blockage of arteries). When arteries supplying the brain are blocked, a stroke can result. When the blocked arteries are the ones which supply the heart, a heart attack can result. High blood pressure alone can cause a blood vessel to burst. The kidneys can be damaged as well. The problem is basically cyclical. Atherosclerosis is often referred to as "hardening of the arteries". Since tension causes the blood pressure to rise, materials such as cholesterol are forced into the walls of the arteries. Naturally, as these materials build up, blood flow is further restricted, and the kidneys seek to compensate by releasing a hormone whose job is to increase the blood pressure. Then more materials are forced into the vessel walls and the cycle continues. The kidney areas on the foot should be worked thoroughly. Much of the problem is the alarm reaction and the inability to return to homeostasis. (See pg. 15). The solar plexus is a key to this problem. It is involved in many key areas in the alarm reaction by providing nerve supply as well as muscular contraction of the diaphragm to meet these challenges. Work this area of the foot repeatedly. The adrenal glands are the key endocrine glands for meeting stress, both short and long term. Work their areas thoroughly.
A deficiency of sugar in the blood. There are many interrelated systems that keep this level constant, despite large changes in the consumption or expulsion of glucose (blood sugar). All carbohydrates are converted to glucose. Glucose is stored in the form of glycogen in the liver and muscles. When glucose is needed it is removed from the glycogen storehouses. A variety of exotic hormones maintain the balance between the combustion of glucose and its storage. Insulin is the most important hormone in this process (See Diabetes). Hypoglycemia is characterized by too much insulin in the blood. It removes glucose from the blood by increasing combustion, and thus increases the amount of glycogen in storage. This is at the expense of the blood. There are many symptoms of hypoglycemia. Sudden drops in energy levels and mental depression are often signs of this disorder. It can impair the efficiency of the brain which depends on a constant supply of blood sugar because it has no stores of its own. Careful working of the pancreas areas on both right and left feet is necessary. The adrenal glands are involved because of their regulation of the storage of proteins, carbohydrates, and fats. The liver is a storehouse and regulator for glycogen. The thyroid and pituitary play a role in metabolism and therefore are involved in this process. Working all the endocrine glands is helpful.

DISORDER	QUICK REFERENCE	
Infertility		
Male	Testes (pp.52-53)	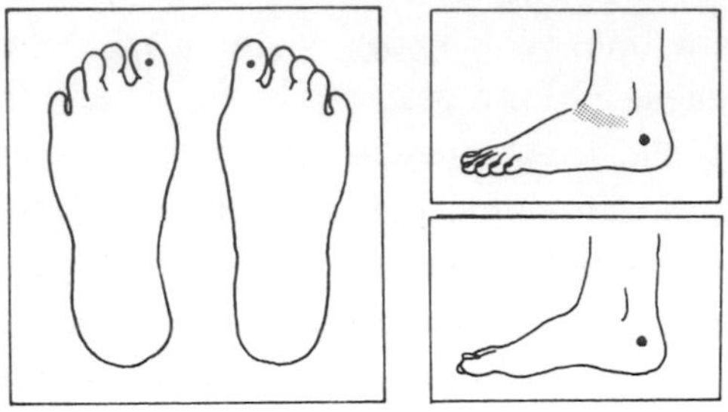
	Prostate (pp.52-53)	
Female	Uterus (pp.52-53)	
	Ovaries (pp.52-53)	
	Fallopian Tubes (p. 51)	
	Pituitary (p. 30)	
Kidney Disorders	Kidney (pp.40-42,44)	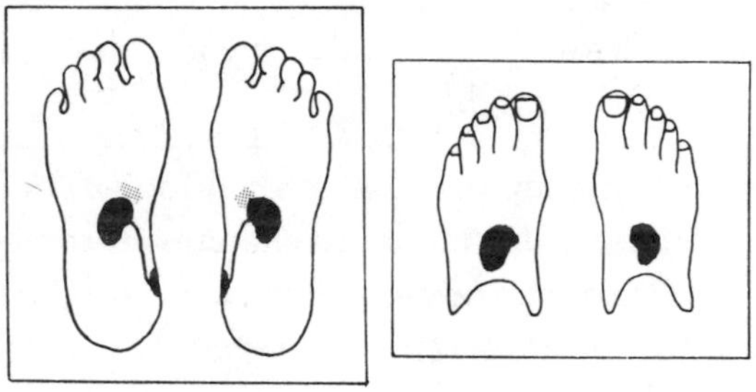
	Ureter Tubes (p. 45)	
	Bladder (pp.47-48)	
	Adrenal Glands (with infection) (pp.40-42)	
Kidney Stones	Kidneys (pp.40-42,44)	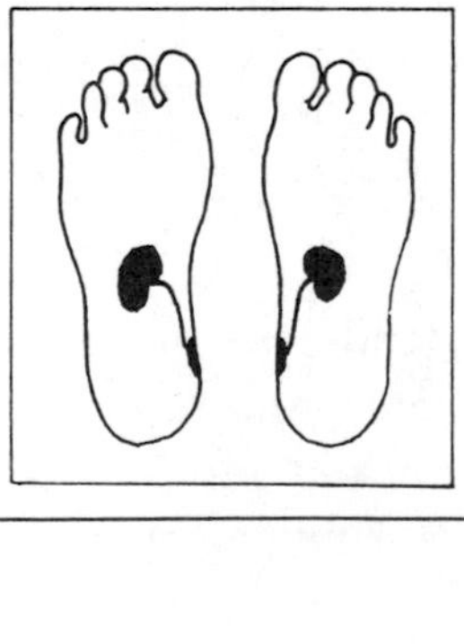
	Ureter Tubes (p. 45)	
	Bladder (pp.47-48)	
Lower Back *See*	*Back* *Hip Disorders* *Sciatica*	

DESCRIPTION AND EMPHASIS
The inability to conceive a child because of structural, endocrine gland, or psychological problems. Infertility requires a team effort. Both partners are to be considered, unless a professional diagnosis has already pointed to the source of the problem. In the female (See Female Disorders) a number of malfunctions of the egg producing mechanism and transport system can occur. The fallopian tubes may be blocked for example. In some cases working the pituitary area on each big toe has proven beneficial in normalizing the monthly ovulation cycle. At times emotions are a factor. Expectation and worry may contribute to the overall imbalances in the systems. The solar plexus area (as a key to tension) needs emphasis. Another possibility is that the male is not producing enough sperm to cause conception. Thus the testicle and prostate areas need emphasis. The rest of the endocrine glands are interrelated with the reproductive functions. Work them thoroughly for any reproductive dysfunction.
The most common disorders involve the kidneys filtration function. The nephrons or little filters (of which there are about a million in the kidneys) can become infected. The flow of urine can be obstructed. The ureter tubes can be blocked by stones (see kidney stones), pressure from other organs and enlargement of the prostate (in men). The urine can become stagnated and can carry infection which leads to serious damage. The kidneys can be damaged by hypertension. (See Hypertension) Edema or excessive accumulation of fluids in the body is at times caused by kidney disease (See pg. 100). Many conditions can cause edema. The kidneys, however, should always be worked to eliminate this excess. Toxicity in the body can be assisted by working the kidneys. The toxins are a by-product of cell metabolism. The kidneys, as chief eliminator can filter the blood disposing of the waste.
Kidney stones occur when the urine is too concentrated. Various substances such as calcium salts, uric acid and other materials crystalize. They can pass out without notice when they are small. However if they become large, the sensitive ureter tubes can be affected. The ureters are elastic but as the large kidney stones try to pass out, their jagged edges catch on the narrow sensitive walls. Surgery may become necessary to remove them. Whatever the situation, the kidneys, ureters and bladder areas on the feet need careful attention.

DISORDER	QUICK REFERENCE	
Lump in Breast *See* *Breast*		
Lung Disorders *See* *Asthma* *Emphysema*		
Menopause *See* *Female Disorders*		
Menstruation *See* *Female Disorders*		
Migraine *See* *Headaches*		
Neck *See* *Back*		
Numbness in the Fingertips	The 7th Cervical (p. 31) Solar Plexus (p. 36)	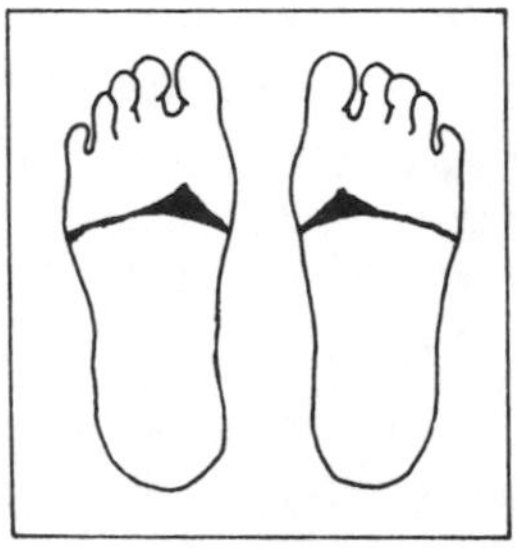 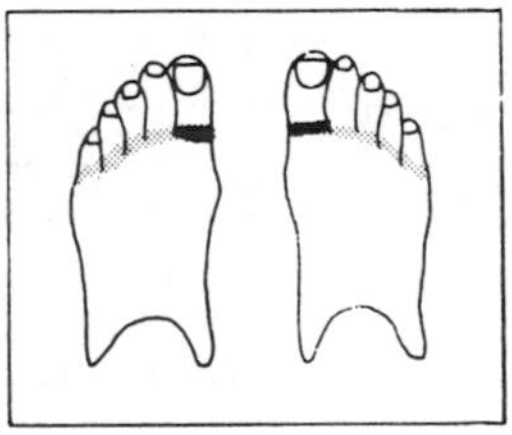
Paralysis	Entire body Neck (pp.32-34) Spine (pp.47-48) Top of Head (p. 32)	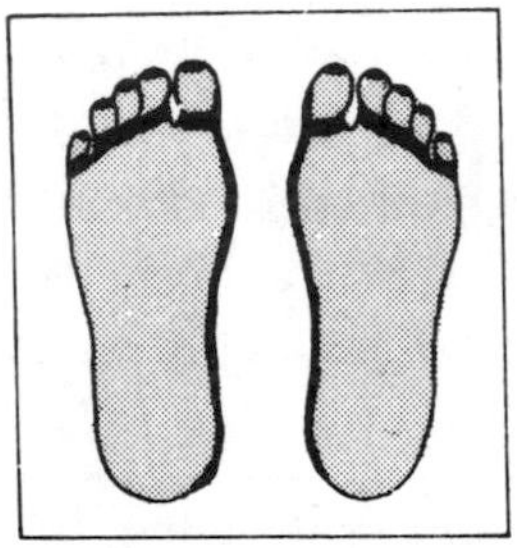
Phlebitis	Liver (pp.40-42) Adrenal Glands (pp.40-42)	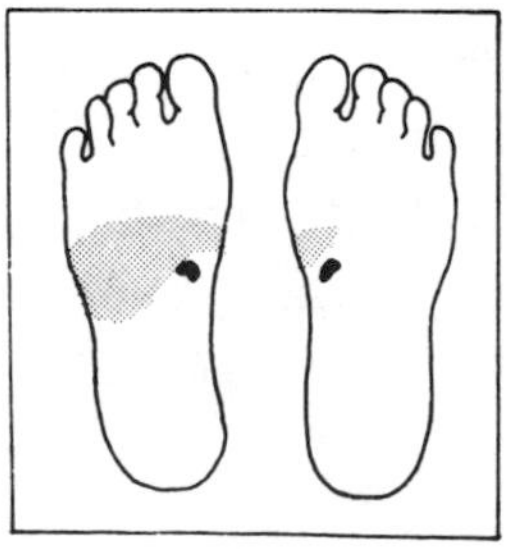

DESCRIPTION AND EMPHASIS
The seventh cervical can affect everything from the base of the neck down into the finger-tips. The cervical vertebrae are vulnerable to tension. Tension in the solar plexus area can lead to tension in the neck. Concentrate on the seventh cervical and the solar plexus areas of the feet.
Paralysis has many causes (i.e., stroke, injury, etc.). The sooner after the incident the person is reached the better chance there is for corrective intervention. New findings have shown that paralyzed limbs can be worked with beneficial results, despite nerve damage and loss of sensitivity. The entire body, including arms, legs, hands and feet, should be worked for general circulation. Paralysis requires extreme dedication because of a variety of factors: the victim's age, the length of time since the injury, and the extent of the damage, all of which influence the outcome of treatment. The chance of success is unknown at this time and requires further study.
An inflammation usually associated with blockage of a vein by a blood clot. The liver is involved in the clotting mechanism and is a helpful area to work on the feet. The part of the arm corresponding to the affected part of the leg (referral area) is a valuable tool for reaching the problem. DO NOT WORK on the affected area itself. Working the adrenal glands helps with the inflammation.

DISORDER	QUICK REFERENCE
Prostate Disorders	Prostate (pp.52-53) Testicle (pp.52-53) Lymph/Groin (p. 51) Lower Back/Bladder (pp.48-50) 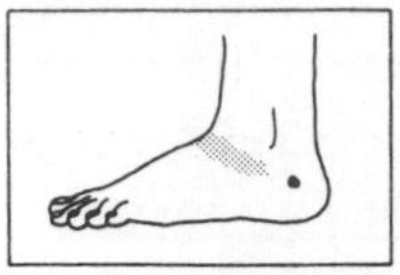 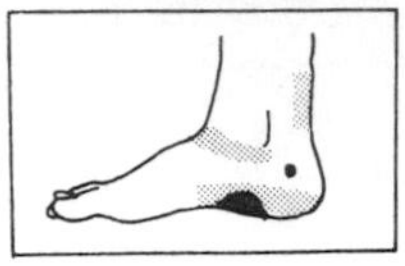
Psoriasis	Kidneys (pp.40-42,44) Thyroid (p. 31) Adrenal Glands (pp.40-42) Pituitary (p. 30) 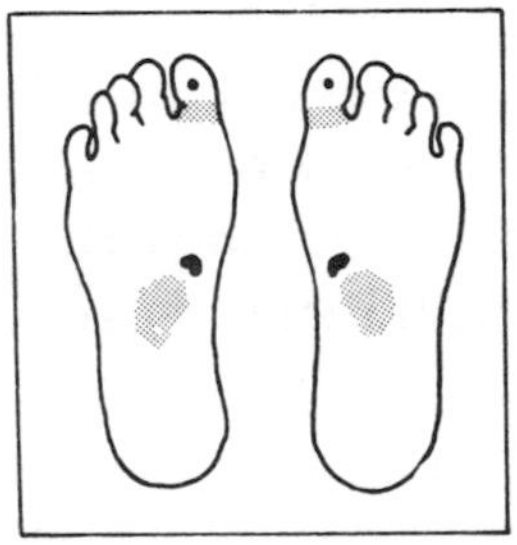
Reproductive Disorders *See* *Female Disorders*, *Infertility*, *Prostate Disorders*	
Rheumatism *See* *Arthritis*, *Bursitis*	
Ringing in the Ears *See* *Tinnitis*	
Sciatica	Hip/Sciatic (p. 49) Lymphatic/Groin (p. 51) Lower Back/Tailbone (pp.47-48) Knee/Leg (p. 50) 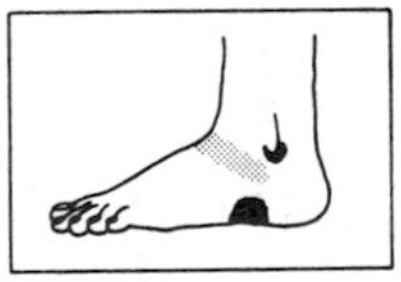 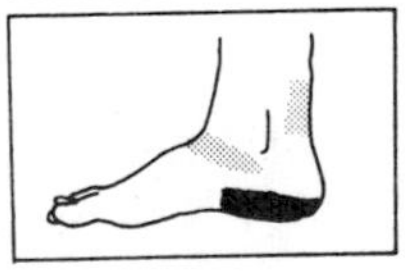
Sciatica *See Also* *Back*	

DESCRIPTION AND EMPHASIS
A male gland behind the outlet of the bladder surrounding the urethra. It contributes the thin, milky alkaline fluid to the semen. The prostate will enlarge due to disease or injury, causing the continued urge to urinate with some discomfort. This is common in middle-aged to older men. Work the prostate/uterus area on the feet. For extra emphasis walk your thumb (See below) down the inside of the leg on the underside about mid-calf to ankle bone. The rest of the reproductive and lower back areas should be worked.
A disorder of the outer layer of skin. It typically looks like thickened red blotches with a scaley surface, mostly affecting the scalp, back and arms. In normal skin, old cells form the outer layer of skin and new cells are formed underneath. In psoriasis, the situation is accelerated, with new cells being formed before the old cells can be shed. The endocrine glands, particularly the thyroid and adrenal glands, contribute to this process. The kidney, as chief eliminator of the body, takes some of the burden off the skin (which also eliminates waste products).
A common term for a persistant pain around the sciatic nerve. The sciatic nerve is the largest nerve in the body. It branches from the lower back down both legs and branches again above the knee. From the knee it stirrups around the heel. The pain is a symptom. But the reason for most sciatic pain is pressure on a spinal nerve by a slipped disc. Direct pressure (i.e. from a poor seating position) is a less common cause for this pain. The hip/sciatic area needs thorough coverage. The inside of the leg on the underside of the bone can be used in addition to the hip/sciatic area of the feet. A great deal of buildup can be encountered at the junction of the lymphatic groin area and the top of the ankle bone where the hip sciatic makes an upper loop. The lower back/tailbone area and the bottom of the heel should be emphasized. Working the knee/leg area can benefit this problem as well.

DISORDER	QUICK REFERENCE	
Shoulder Disorders	Shoulder (pp.37-39) Neck (pp.32-34) Mid Back (pp.48-50) Arm Area (p. 43)	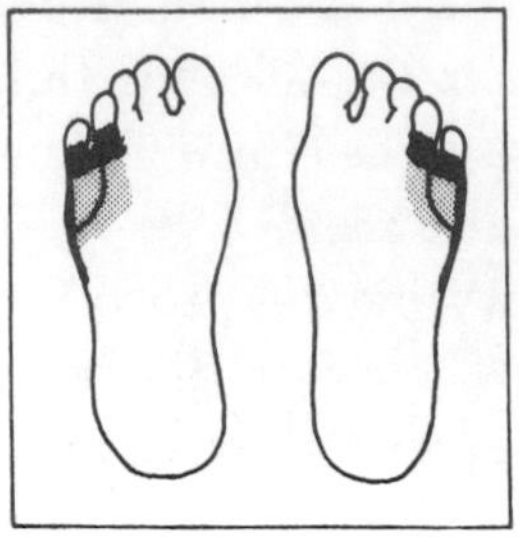
Shoulder Disorders	*See Also Bursitis*	
Sinusitis	Head/Neck/Sinus (pp.32-34) Ileocecal Valve (pp.44-45) Adrenal Glands (pp.40-42) Pituitary (p. 30)	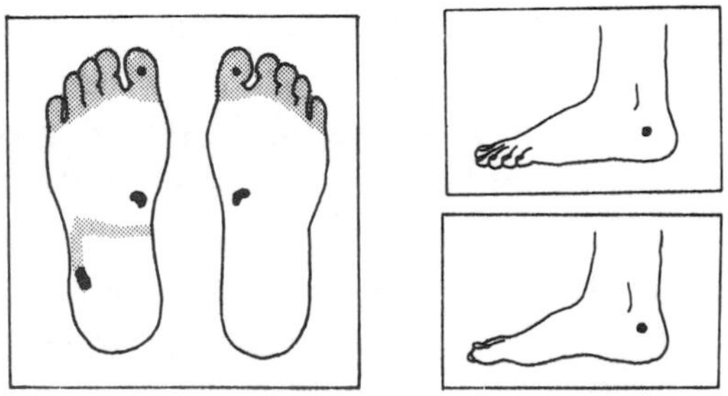
Skin Disorders	Kidney (pp. 40-42, 44) Thyroid (p. 31) Reproductive Glands (pp. 52-53) Adrenal Glands (pp. 40-42) Pituitary (p. 30)	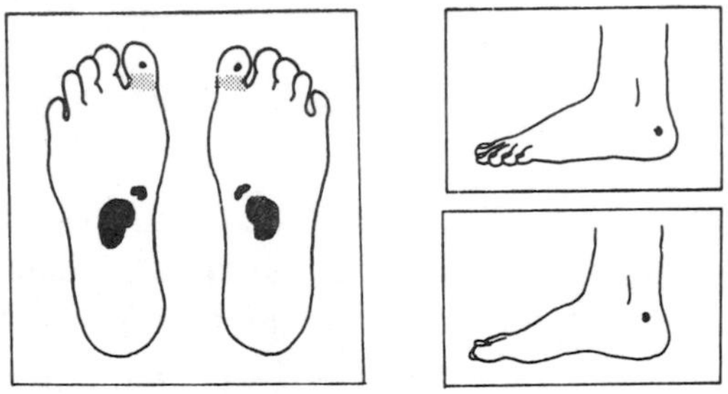
Skin Disorders	*See Also Eczema* *Psoriasis*	
Sore Throat	Neck (pp.32-34) Adrenal Glands (pp.40-42) Lymphatic Area (p. 51)	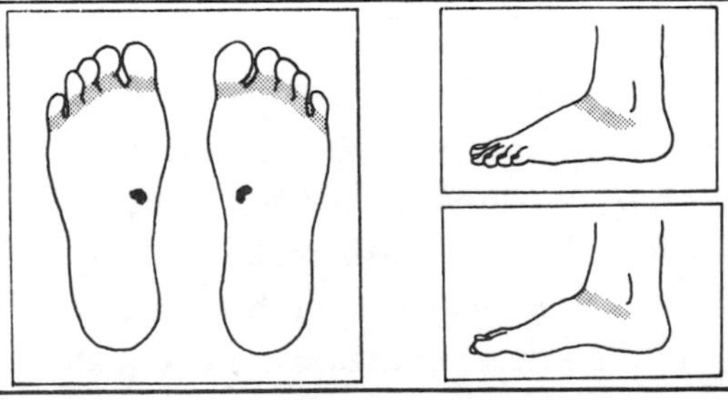

DESCRIPTION AND EMPHASIS
Pain in the shoulder can come from areas outside the shoulder region. The neck and mid-back region are helper areas for this problem. Work the shoulder areas on the top and bottom of feet. The neck areas should be thoroughly covered. Tenderness will frequently be encountered in the midback area. The arm area can provide additional help. Corns and callouses are frequently associated with this problem because of their ability to block the zone (pg. 19).
Sinuses are hollow cavities lined with thin membranes throughout the head region. Mucus coats these membranes to protect them. The only known anatomical function of the sinuses is to resonate the voice. The sinus cavities can become clogged with excessive mucus causing headaches and congestion. When the cavities become infected the condition is called sinusitis. All the toes need careful attention on all sides, top and bottom. The ileocecal valve is an important area for this problem. The valve is a passageway between the small and large intestines for control of the flow of wastes. The area around the ileocecal valve has a great deal of influence on the mucus level in the body.
The skin is considered an organ. Its disorders attract more attention than those of a similar magnitude affecting other organs. The skin is one of the bodys eliminators. Improper elimination can blemish the skin. The functioning of the kidneys and endocrine glands are important. Areas of emphasis depend on the type of disorder. Acne requires emphasis of the reproductive and the pituitary areas. Dry skin or oily skin involves the thyroid and pituitary.
The area of infection in the throat can be found in the feet by carefully searching the tops, bottoms, and sides of the toes. Always work the adrenal glands for infections.

DISORDER	QUICK REFERENCE	
Stroke	Top of Head (p. 32) Head (pp.32-34) Spine (pp.47-48)	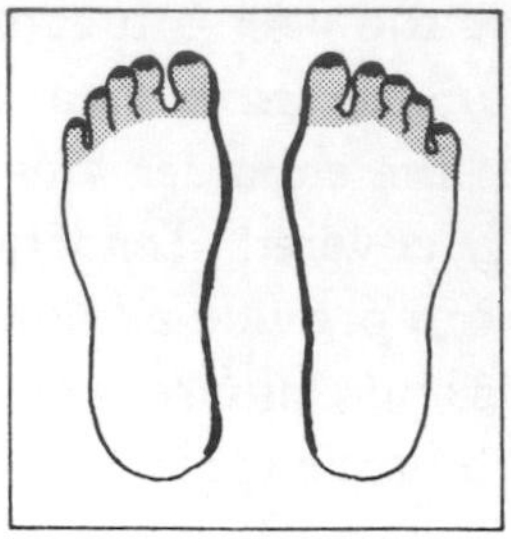
Stroke *See Also*	*Heart Attack* *Hypertension* *Paralysis*	
Tinnitis	Eye/Ear (pp.35-36) Neck (pp.32-34) Adrenal Glands (pp.40-42)	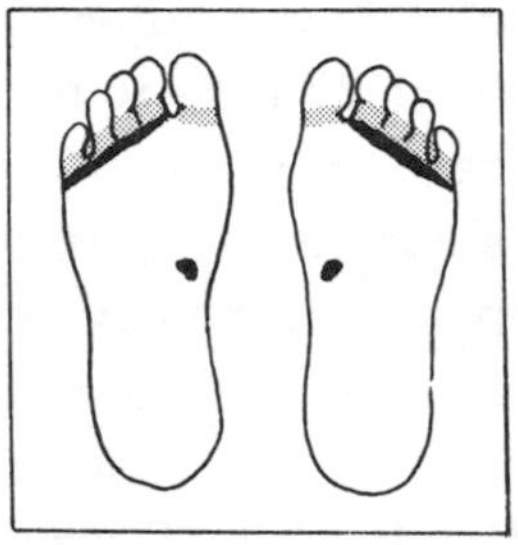
Tinnitis *See Also*	*Hearing Disorders*	
Tailbone Disorders *See*	*Back (Tailbone) Disorders*	
Tendonitis *See*	*Bursitis*	
Tonsillitis	Lymphatic (p. 51) Neck (pp.32-34) Adrenal Glands (pp.40-42)	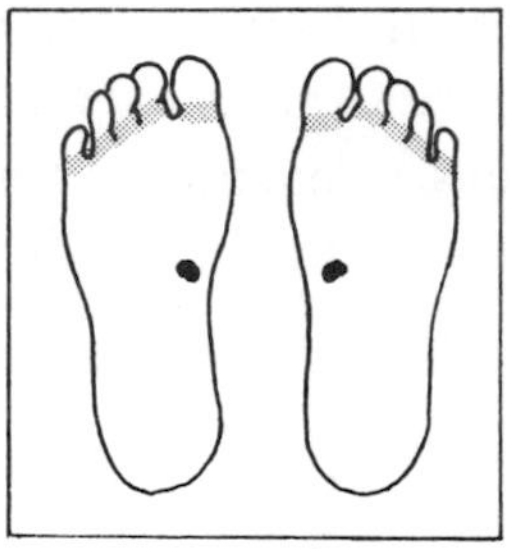 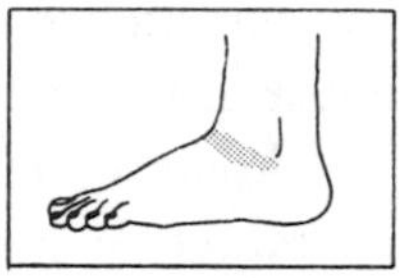 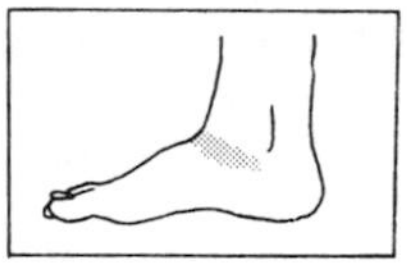
Tumors	Pituitary (p. 30) Corresponding Area	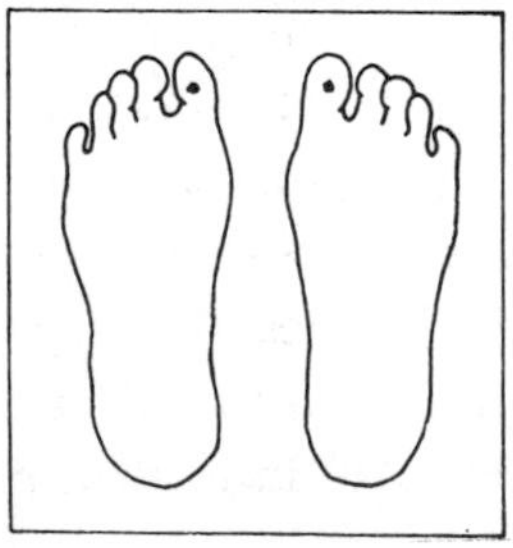

DESCRIPTION AND EMPHASIS
A sudden rupture or clotting of a blood vessel in the brain. Work the top of the head area on the big toe opposite the side of the stroke. Try the tops of the smaller toes also. The entire head/neck/sinus and spine areas should be worked.
A ringing, buzzing, or hissing in the ear. It can arise from any disorder of the ear or of the auditory nerve. Wax in the ear, blockage of the Eustachian tube, and irritation of the auditory nerve are the most common causes. Work the eye/ear and neck areas completely. The adrenal gland area is worked for possible infection in the Eustachian tube.
An infection in the throat of the mass lymphoid tissue called the tonsils. Work the lymphatic area, the neck area, and the adrenal gland area for infection. Search the bottom of the toe as the stem goes into the ball of the toe and work it thoroughly.
Any swelling or enlargement, particularly a growth which performs no particular function. The pituitary gland controls the growth of soft and hard tissue in the body. It controls not only how big a person grows but can affect the growth of tumors. Tumors can be cancerous. Basically cancer is a breakdown in the orderly rate of growth of the cells. The result is a puzzling array of diseases. In addition to the pituitary, the area corresponding to the tumor should be explored. Use the zones to find this area on the foot.

DISORDER	QUICK REFERENCE	
Varicose Veins	Colon (pp.44-46) Endocrine Glands (pp.40-42, 52-53)	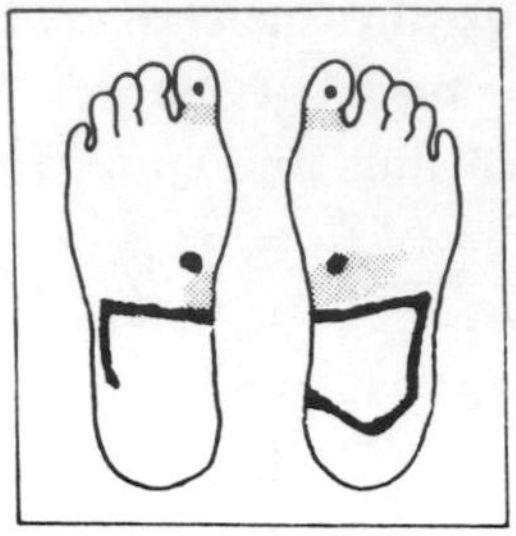
Vertigo *See Dizziness*		
Ulcer Ulcer *See Also*	Stomach (if affected) (pp.40-42) Solar Plexus (p. 36) Diaphragm (p. 36) Adrenals (pp.40-42) *Hypertension*	
Urinary Disorders or Infection *See*	*Bladder Disorders* *Kidney Disorders* *Prostate Disorders*	
Whiplash **Whiplash** *See*	Neck (pp.32-34) Lung (pp.37-39) Spine (pp.47-48) *Back (Cervicals)*	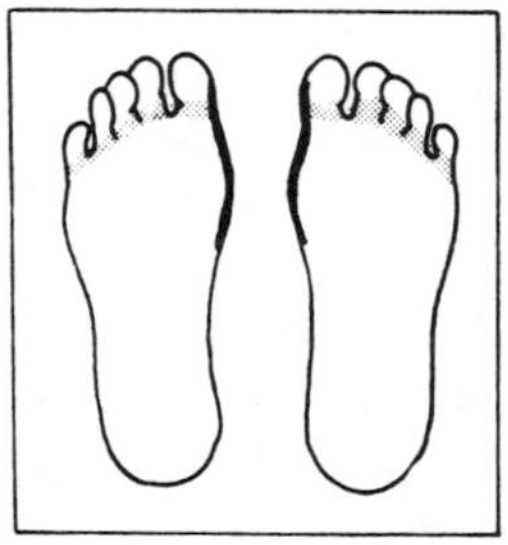 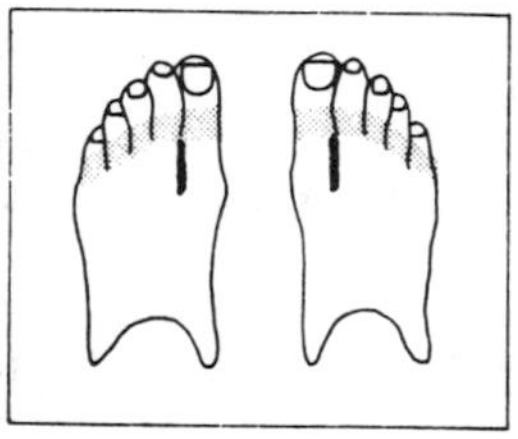

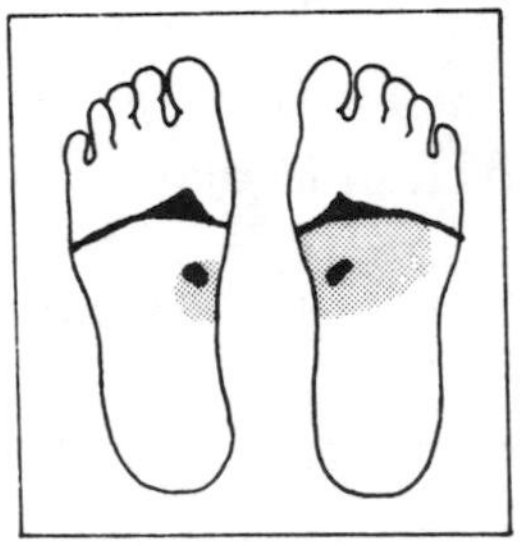

DESCRIPTION AND EMPHASIS
Blue veins in the legs usually caused by abnormal swelling. Blood moves in the veins by muscular pressure of the legs on the blood vessels. A series of one way valves ensures that the flow is upward. If the valves are defective the blood stagnates, the pressure builds and the veins can become swollen and painful. Pressure can be caused by problems in the colon, excessive standing, tumors or anything else that puts strain on the system. The corresponding area on the arm can be helpful (See pg. 12). The endocrine glands, particularly the adrenal glands, have an affect on the vessels of circulation.
A persistent break in the skin or mucus membrane that fails to heal. Circulation is not functioning in the area. There are many types and locations of ulcers, the most common of which is in the stomach. The solar plexus can help with stress related disorders, although not all ulcers are associated with stress. Working the adrenal glands helps with stress as well as assisting with the inflammation. Work the stomach area on the feet.
A sprain of the muscles and tendons of the back of the neck caused by a sudden blow from the rear, such as when the rear of one's automobile is smashed into. This damage is not simply located around the 7th cervical. It extends down the thoracic vertebrae. The muscles and tendons through the upper back are frequently involved. The first and second zones are of particular importance. Work the neck area in all the toes. Cover the spine area thoroughly. Work down the first and second zone between the big toe and the next toe in the lung area.

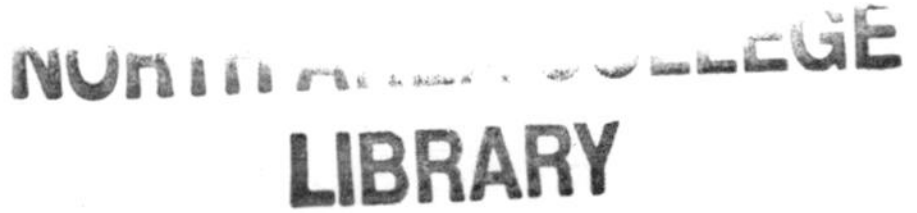

Postscript

Once you have mastered the techniques and have developed your treatment pattern, you are bound to start thinking about other things. Since the goal is not to become "mechanical" in your approach, you should allow your intuition and spontaneity to take over. Compare it to learning to play a musical instrument. You practice the techniques, the scales; you study the theory. But music is more than this. You must be able to develop a *sense* of the work, a *feeling* for it. You do the same thing with each pair of feet. This is what makes reflexology the engrossing and fulfilling study it is.

The key is observation. The more feet you work on, the more familiar you will become with slight irregularities and unusual conditions in them. You will probably catch yourself comparing each foot to the others in a mental monologue, like "Hmmmm, this big toe doesn't feel like the last one." This is fine. It is a sign that you are arriving. You will develop definite patterns in your work. They will vary from problem to problem.

So, what makes a good reflexologist? More than anything else it is hard work and perseverance. Reflexology just is not suited to anyone looking for fast solutions with minimal effort. It takes time and dedication, a persistent approach to the daily challenges to our health.

How do you find a good reflexologist? What do you look for? Chapter 4 ("You the Reflexologist") gives some excellent guidelines. Of course you don't want someone who promises to cure specific illnesses, who prescribes for illness, or who diagnoses your problems. Reflexologists are not trained in these matters and it is not within the scope of reflexology to perform these services.

Avoid the "mechanics" too. These are the ones who have discovered that a great deal of pressure can be applied using a wild assortment of instruments and knuckles. It is a lazy and dangerous approach and it is NOT a part of reflexology. This does not include the practitioner who recommends rollers or other self-help techniques that you use on yourself, so that *you* can gauge *your own* pressure.

You're not looking for a foot massage. There is nothing wrong with a good foot massage but it is not reflexology. If you find yourself in the care of a "reflexologist" who uses oils to give your feet a general rubdown, seek out another practitioner. But applying cream AFTER the treatment is within the bounds of acceptable practice.

If your reflexologist uses extreme pressure without regard for your tolerance level, ask him or her to desist. Explain that you expect a more sensitive approach. If you don't get it, find another reflexologist. In many cases the practitioner can alter his or her style to suit your needs. Have patience, but don't put yourself through a lot of pain and discomfort. Remember, that you are there for relaxation. If you don't feel relaxed after the treatment, talk it over with your reflexologist. It will help him or her establish the appropriate level of pressure for YOUR feet.

The same is true of nail gouging. Always tell your reflexologist if you feel a finger or thumb nail hitting your foot. If it continues, there is something seriously wrong with his or her technique and you may have to look for another reflexologist. Remember that it is up to you to evaluate your reflexologist, to be sure you're getting what you came for. That's what this book has been designed to help you do. A reflexologist, for example, who pays attention to your comments or signals gets high marks and deserves a second chance.

Since reflexology is a grassroots movement, you should not be concerned about appearances and amenities. What is most important is that your reflexologist applies the techniques properly, evaluates your feet carefully, and responds to you in a way that satisfies YOU. If YOU'RE not happy, look for someone else. And for those of you who are or will become reflexologists, once you have identified the kind of practitioner you want for your own feet you will see the kind of reflexologist that you should strive to be.

INDEX